Dying With Open Eyes

Dying With Open Eyes

✦

Alzheimer's Disease

Jennie Swanson Dincecco

iUniverse, Inc.
New York Lincoln Shanghai

Dying With Open Eyes
Alzheimer's Disease

Copyright © 2005 by Jennie Swanson Dincecco

iUniverse books may be ordered through booksellers or by contacting:

iUniverse
2021 Pine Lake Road, Suite 100
Lincoln, NE 68512
www.iuniverse.com
1-800-Authors (1-800-288-4677)

Cover Design by Laurie Swanson Kiesewetter

ISBN: 0-595-34054-7 (pbk)
ISBN: 0-595-67057-1 (cloth)

Printed in the United States of America

Dedicated
with love
to

Dick
who stood by and with me
and is with me yet

And to

Laurie, Jeff, Scott, Bruce, Kim, Ryan,
Blake, Jamie, Kristin, Kelsey,
and Mollie
who helped to put me together again

And to

Bill, Barb, Vito, Margie, Brooke, Athy, Joan,
Virginia, Jini, and Don,
who led me back into the world

And to

The Reagan family and the Shriver family for their courage in sharing their pain
and caring

And to

To the Alzheimer's Association for help and hope

And to

Ruby, Marge, and my fellow caregivers

And to

Tom

My life's reward for loving

STORMS MAKE TREES TAKE DEEPER ROOTS

—Claude McDonald

Contents

List of Illustrations

Acknowledgements

To

The Harvard University Press
for permission
To
reprint the poems of
Emily Dickinson

And to
The President of
the Alzheimer's Association
who has "been there"

And to
Lloene Martin
Of Trainman Productions
For permission to reprint the words to
Winds of Yesterday

And to
Agnes Hoepker and Ron Amack, my iUniverse coordinators
for their guidance

And to

Scott, Bruce, and Roger
for their computer expertise and help

And to

Laurie for the cover design, to Jeff for encouragement and computer use

And to

Tom for help in editing and for love and support

Introduction

I initially wrote this book as therapy for myself as a caregiver for my Mom who had Alzheimer's disease. Mom wanted me to make a record of the experience. She had been a teacher most of her life and she knew the value of a shared experience. Mom's wish was that I share her story to help others, so all proceeds of this book go to the Alzheimer's Association in support of their vision of a world without Alzheimer's disease. Mom gave me permission for this book during the early stage of the disease. We both understood that she would have no control over the disease and its attendant indignities. However, Mom would would always be treated with well-deserved dignity.

My jottings kept me company during Mom's night wanderings. They caused me to be more aware of my surroundings and heightened my senses. They forced me to face my challenges. They showed me the changes in myself. They filled many lonely hours as I sat by Mom's bedside and slowly began to realize the benefits of caregiving. They are a part of me, a legacy to my children and grandchildren.

The jottings also demonstrated my search for current information and the relentless decline of a person with Alzheimer's disease.

> If a sudden death hits like an explosion,
> Knocking you flat, then a slow decline
> Arrives like a glacier, massive and
> Unstoppable, grinding you down.
>
> —Edward Myers, 1983
> *When Parents Die*

My wish is that this book will give hope to other caregivers. According to Vaclav Havel in *Disturbing the Peace: A Conversation with Karel Huizdala*, "Hope is not the conviction that something will turn out well, but the certainty that something makes sense regardless of how it turns out".

As I became less absorbed in the daily therapy of journal writing, I became more concerned with the bigger picture of Alzheimer's disease. Dr. Roses, Chief of the Joseph and Kathleen Bryan Alzheimer's Disease Research Center at Duke University Medical Center in Durham, N.C., argues that their research findings may support the long-held hypothesis that Alzheimer's disease is something that eventually occurs in all human beings. Carrying a certain gene (E4) may simply mean that you get the disease earlier. Dr. John E. Morley, Chief of Geriatric Medicine at the St. Louis School of Medicine states, "Given that most of us are going to get Alzheimer's disease instead of AIDS, the investment (going into research) is well worth it."

After my experience with Alzheimer's disease, I realize that there is an area of research which needs more public exposure and funding. The disease is a brain disease and research on the brain of Alzheimer's victims may help unlock the mystery of cause and cure. Many caretakers are not aware of the value of a brain autopsy after death or of the procedures to arrange for an autopsy for research purposes. I wasn't aware. Furthermore, the autopsy must be completed under standard scientific conditions to be considered adequate research. Often these research protocols are available only at major medical centers.

Caregivers can contribute in a significant way to research by making arrangements for a brain autopsy prior to the death of their loved one. The autopsy should take place at an institution doing research on Alzheimer's disease.

I also learned that my field of study for my Doctorate in Human Growth and Development was helpful to me as a caregiver. I was familiar with normal growth and development of infants and children as well as adults. I wrote a book with Dr. Leonard Kise on growth and development for parents called Partners in Child Development. The knowledge of growth and development patterns, as well as my teaching experiences in regular and special education, and my research background, helped me as I watched my Mom reverse and sometimes distort the normal developmental patterns. My experiences as a Director of a Nursery School and, later, as the Director of Early Childhood Education in a public school system, gave me some practical ways of caring for Mom as she exhibited a reversal of some of the normal developmental milestones of childhood. I also realized that even though the developmental milestones were similar, an adult has a lifetime of experiences which should be respected. When we interact with adults who have Alzheimer's disease, we should always be respectful of the person's dignity.

The poems of Emily Dickinson were meaningful to me. They inspired me. They gave me a reason to think about an issue in a different way. I have included one or more of her poems in each chapter where I thought they might be relevant and meaningful to caregivers. The punctuation and capitalizations are as Emily Dickinson wrote them. She did not give titles to the poems. The chapter titles are not titles for the poems. They are simply chapter titles.

The chapters are short because I found, as a caregiver, that it was difficult to concentrate or to have time to read.

I hope that other caregivers find, as I did after the caregiving experience, a sense of satisfaction and peace and a new understanding and appreciation of their own humanity.

Finally, I have thought about the musings of Henry David Thoreau in his journal, "How vain it is to sit down when you have not stood up to live." I have lived and want to write about it. I do as Thoreau suggests, "Say what you have to say, not what you ought. Any truth is better than make believe."
This is my truth.

Jennie Swanson Dincecco
Woodstock, Illinois

1

The Promise of Life is Death

Suspense-is Hostiler than Death-
Death-tho'soever Broad,
Is just Death, and cannot increase-
Suspense-does not conclude-

But perishes-to live anew-
But just anew to die
Annihilation-plated fresh
With Immortality-

—Emily Dickinson, 1863

It is 2 A.M. in a small South Georgia town. Dad gets out of bed and shuffles down the hall. He sits in his favorite chair and has a massive heart attack. He dies instantly. It is just that quick. At the same time, Mom is awakened by a peculiar silence and finds Dad slumped over in his chair. He passed from life to death suddenly. That's the way death is for some people. For others, death is like a late night visitor who keeps saying "Goodnight" but doesn't leave.

Lack of predictability and helplessness were the things that Dad feared. He was a railroad man. When trains were on time, life was predictable and he felt a sense of control. He would reach into his vest pocket and pull out his gold watch which was attached to a long gold chain. He would note that it was 10:36 and the 10:38 train was pulling into the station. He would "grin like a chessie cat" and nod his head in satisfaction.

Mom was always the one who could handle "those times," the times when things were out of control. They became a challenge to her. Mom and Dad had been married for 53 years. They had known good and hard times. Mostly, there were good times.

On this night though, Mom is awakened by the silence in their bedroom. Dad's snoring had become a part of the familiar night noises. Tonight, every-thing is quiet. She calls, "Ches." No answer. She calls louder.

The light is on in the bathroom and the door is open. Mom sits on the edge of the bed for a few moments. It is still silent. She brushes her graying hair off of her face and pads slowly down the hall.

The silence makes her heart begin to throb. She is more awake than ever now. Her eyes dart from side to side on the lookout for any surprises. She wipes the perspiration from her nose, hitches up her nightgown, and moves quickly from the bathroom to the kitchen.

She sees Dad sitting slumped over in his favorite chair. She slowly rubs the back of his neck and calls to him. No answer. There is silence. She picks up his hand. It seems cold and heavy. She cries out, "Oh, Lord." The silence is over, broken by bleeding tears and racking sobs.

The sirens on the ambulance pierce the silence of the cool night air for a few minutes. The hospital is only blocks away. Everything is only blocks away in this little town.

The paramedics ask Mom to step back. They all know Dad and Mom. They ask a few questions of Mom, check on Dad's vital signs, and quickly put him on the stretcher and into the ambulance. They hoist Mom into the seat next to the stretcher.

Upon arrival at the hospital, the doctors review Dad's medical history. Dad had been in excellent health until 1971 when he had several transient ischemic attacks. These are brief interruptions of the blood supply to a part of the brain which results in a temporary impairment. After one of these attacks, Dad had dif-ficulty talking and using his right arm. He underwent several tests and the diag-nosis was cerebral vascular disease. He was placed on medication and did well until his seventy-ninth year when he had an acute myocardial infarction, a heart attack. He was then transferred to another city where he had surgery to open a clogged carotid artery. That was four years ago. Since then, Dad has been enjoy-ing his garden, reading news magazines, talking with friends, fishing, and being with his family. At the time of his fatal heart attack, he was eighty-three years old.

During those last four years, Dad found the time for his two special interests, storytelling about his railroad days and writing. He told us the railroad stories over and over, complete with poems and songs. His writings were mostly about his life and what he had learned from his varied experiences. Little did we know that he was creating a family history for generations yet unborn.

One of his writings was labeled, Memo 1899-1979:

Reflections on next August 19th caused me to stop and briefly review what's been happening to me over the past 80 years. The most important event was when Cleo and I joined hands and married on February 5th, 1930, and later were joined by Sonny and Sister in our march down life's highway together. They brought us much happiness and it was great to observe our four grand-children develop, bringing us many additional pleasures and much content-ment. I have owned three homes, several cars, have never been arrested, and have given lots and lots of advice and took some. At one point, I had an inferi-ority complex, perhaps due to not finishing high school. I grew up during the Great Depression, and this, plus the serious illness of my Dad for years, explains that. But, as time went by and, after I had attended college night school for several years, more and more people with college degrees showed up as competition, and they seemed to have no more sense than I thought I had, so out went the inferiority complex. So what lessons have I learned? What truths have been discovered? What wisdom gained?

I have never made a lot of money even though my family always lived com-fortably. I have never been president of my company and am not sure that my life has been a great success. However, if happiness is a criterion, the answer is an unequivocal "Yes." I say this as I always loved my family, as well as enjoyed the nearly 50 years I was associated with the fine folks with the Express Com-pany.

Finally, I simply cannot visualize anyone being more contented and happy, and I would surely not change a thing.

Ches

These were the words of a person who came of age in the Depression era. They were also the words of Mom's life companion. His sudden death signaled the traumatic beginning of Mom's unraveling.

2

Sudden Death

There's been a Death, in the Opposite House,
As Lately as Today-
I know it, by the numb look
Such Houses have-always-

The Neighbors rustle in and out-
The Doctor-drives away-
A Window opens like a Pod-
Abrupt-mechanically-

Somebody flings a Mattress out-
The Children hurry by-
They wonder if it died-on that-
I used to-when a Boy-

The Minister-goes stiffly in-
As if the House were His-
And He owned all the Mourners-now-
And little Boys-besides-

And then the Milliner-and the Man
Of the Appalling Trade-
To take the measure of the House-

There'll be that Dark Parade-

Of Tassels-and of Coaches-soon-
It's easy as a Sign-

The Intuition of the News-
In just a Country Town-

—Emily Dickinson, 1862

Dad's last words flood Mom's mind as she sits waiting for the doctor who is an old family friend. He weeps with Mom as he shares the news of Dad's death. He calls it a sudden death. There is no time to say, "Goodbye."

Mom is surrounded by friends and family. She is hugged, patted, consoled, listened to, and cared for at the hospital. She is in shock from the sudden death of her life partner of 53 years. Her sobs come from deep within.

Suddenly, she sits upright and says, "I have to call Sonny and Sister." Sonny is my brother and I am Sister.

"Hello." I say sleepily from thousands of miles away.

"Sister, I have some bad news. Dad just died of a heart attack."

"Oh, no." I sit up quickly.

"He got up from bed in the middle of the night and went to his favorite chair; the red leather one, sat down and died."

There was silence and then sobs on both ends of the call.

"Just like that, he's gone."

"He said that when he died, he wanted to go quickly."

"I know."

"Mom, are you okay?"

"Not so good." There is silence again and more sobs.

"I'll be there as soon as I can, probably later today."

"Thanks, Sister."

"I love you, Mom."

"I love you, too."

"Bye. Take care of yourself."

"Bye."

I reach over and gently shake Dick, my husband. His snoring sounds to me like a funeral drum roll. With a loud snort, he wakes up.

"What's the matter?"

"Dad just died...a heart attack."

"Oh Honey," he says as he engulfs me in his arms. I feel safe there and sobs shake my body.

I can't believe that Dad is dead. He was always the one who took care of everyone. He was in control, a benevolent manager. He always looked out for all of us.

He protected us. He provided for us, never lavishly, but I could always count on him. Yet, he nudged me gently to be independent. He encouraged me to get as much education as possible. He was willing to do without so that I could go to a university. He said it was an investment in my future. He was so proud when I earned a Bachelor's degree, and later, a Master's and a Doctorate.

I always knew that I couldn't disappoint Dad even if I didn't go to college because he loved me unconditionally. No, he didn't have to tell me he loved me. He showed me with his actions. That's the truest test of love. Yes, actions speak louder. And yes, I'm feeling sorry for myself. I'm going to miss him. Things will never be the same. These thoughts and others are shared with Dick as we sat clutching each other in the early chill of a March Midwestern dawn.

I finally muffle the tears long enough to call our children, all grown now. Of course, the minute they answer, the tears flow again. I feel safe and comfortable expressing my grief to them. They understand.

Then I call the airlines and make reservations for the next flight to Georgia. We will change planes in Atlanta and then rent a car from Macon to drive to Mom and Dad's hometown.

We throw some clothes in a suitcase, take quick showers, and leave for the airport where I call my office to tell them I'm going to my father's funeral and will call them later about plans for returning. I don't ask for permission. Dad taught us how to make decisions based on priorities. Number one priority is your belief system. This includes your faith, morals, principles, and integrity. Number two is your family. Everything else is subservient to these two priorities. I have been in a quandary many times. When I stop and consider my priorities, my way becomes clear.

When Dick and I drive up to my folks' house, there are lots of cars in the driveway and on the street. There are people milling all over the house and yard. Some are walking slowly in the backyard. Others are sitting on the screened porch or on the patio. It is a patio when the car isn't in the carport. We walk up to the house and are greeted warmly with hugs and "Heys."

The ladies from the church have taken over the kitchen and are cleaning, cooking, and answering the phone. Casserole dishes are on the counter and a large jar of "sun tea" is surrounded by ice tea glasses with sprigs of fresh mint. There are eight cakes in all sizes, shapes, and flavors, including Dad's favorite, a yellow cake with caramel frosting.

Then I see Mom. She suddenly looks older and smaller. We sob and hold each other. Dick joins us in a hug. Then we sit down in the old rocking chairs that belonged to my Granny and talk about Dad for hours with family and friends.

This is an important part of the healing process. We find ourselves feeling better. We realize that Dad will live forever in our hearts. The essence of him will never die.

Mom asks me if I will go with her to the funeral home to make "arrangements." This will be the first time that I have been on the "arranging side" of a funeral. We go into the basement of the funeral home to pick out a casket. Mom says Dad didn't want an expensive casket. He told both of us that when he died, he wanted the economy model.

Yes, Mom and Dad had talked about dying many times in the last few years. Dad even had vaults put in their graves. He also purchased two marble slabs and had his name and Mom's names carved on them. He had made most of the "arrangements." He is still in control. We smile as we remember Dad warmly. Only those who are forgotten are truly gone.

3

Early Signs of Alzheimer's Disease

Mine to stay-when all have wandered-
To devise once more
If the Life be too surrendered-
Life of Mine-restore-

—(Excerpt from Promise This-When You be Dying-)
Emily Dickinson, 1862

It is almost a year since Dad died. The phone rings.

"Jennie, is that you?"

"Yes. Louvenia?" The southern accent sounds like my Mom's cousin who lives near Mom.

"How are you, Honey? I'm sorry to bother you, but I thought you ought to know. Your mother isn't doing too well. We just worry about her all the time. I don't think she's eating well and she's getting forgetful."

"Do you think I should come to see her?"

"Oh, Jennie, she'd love it. I know you were here a few months ago but she seems to be failing."

"I appreciate your call, Louvenia. I'll make arrangements to come."

"Y'all take care and come see us when you're here."

I hang up the phone. I wonder what "failing" means. Mom isn't used to being alone. Maybe it's time to ask her to come and live with us. She and Dad had lived in the Chicago area before so it would not be unfamiliar. She would be surrounded by family. Our adult son, Jeff, is still living at home as well as Dick's mother, Helen, since she had surgery for a pacemaker. She has inoperable cancer. She is a little older than Mom, but they might be company for each other since

Dick and I are both working. On second thought, I wonder what happened to our empty nest. Hey, I even have chickens coming back to roost.

Dick and I talk long into the night about the situation. He feels good about the care we are able to give his mother and would welcome my Mom in our home. He laughs and says, "Maybe we could get funding as a nursing home". We both laugh, not realizing the true meaning of nursing home. That would come much later.

I take three vacation days from work and fly for a long weekend to be with Mom. My cousin meets me at the airport and drives me to Mom's home.

I tap lightly on the door. There is no answer. I knock harder. There was still no answer. Then, I pound loudly on the door. I see the drapery move and then the door opens. There she stands. My once robust and ageless mother is thin, gaunt, and old. I hug her. I used to be swallowed up in her hefty bosom hugs. Now, my arms envelop her. She seems to be inches shorter. I have the feeling of protector, not protected, as in days gone by.

We spend the afternoon on the screened porch rocking in those same old rocking chairs of Granny's. The warm Southern sunshine and the smell of spring flowers give me a sense of peace and nostalgia. They are reminders of my early days and summers with my Granny. I picture my Granny rocking in the same chair where my Mom is sitting.

Suddenly, as if with new eyes, I see Mom as my Granny was. She looks like Granny. Her hair has turned gray with some white around the ears. Her eyes are sunken and character lines (wrinkles) accent her face. She wears a freshly starched cotton dress, stockings, and low-heeled shoes. The stockings are a remnant of Southern breeding. Just like Granny.

We catch up on all the news of the family, both up North and down South.

"Are you okay, Mom?"

"Oh, Sister, sometimes I think I'm losing my mind. I'm getting so forgetful. I was reading in Newsweek about a disease called Alzheimer's. I think I have it."

"Oh Mom, everyone gets a little forgetful with age. You're okay."

"You think so?" Mom looked relieved. Since I received my Doctorate, Mom has tended to think I know everything. She, however, is the one with wisdom.

Her comment about Alzheimer's disease is preposterous to me. Mom is a very intelligent lady who went to college, was a teacher and an artist. She had worked as a volunteer to change the lives of slum children. She always read voraciously and was current in world as well as local events. I laugh softly at her comment which means I don't hear her concern. Denial is common for the family.

Mom fixes me a southern dinner. There is fried chicken, turnip greens with pot liquor (the juice from cooking the turnip greens) to soak the cornbread, potato salad, ambrosia (coconut and orange sections), and iced tea with sprigs of mint from the garden. Only a few things go wrong. She burns the cornbread, and the potato salad has no salad dressing in it. She said she forgot. I'm sure that she is just excited that I have come on such short notice.

After dinner, Mom doesn't want to sit on the porch. She closes all the draperies, locks the doors, and we sit in the parlor (the southern word for living room).

"Mom, do you have enough money to live on?"

"Oh, yes, I don't have much, but it's enough. You can look at the books if you want to."

As long as I can remember, Dad kept books on all expenses just like an accountant. In meticulous handwriting, he would write entry dates, bill amounts, payments, and other details. I stand on a chair to reach the books which are high on the closet shelf. They are right where Dad left them. I open the first book. All of the entries are in Dad's handwriting. The last entry next to the car insurance is his. It is the same with other household expenses.

"Mom, these are all entries made by Dad. Do you have another set of books?"

"No, Honey. They're all there."

"Mom, have you paid the car insurance lately?"

"It's all there in the books."

"But, Mom, these entries were all made before Dad died. It's been almost a year.

Have you been paying the bills?"

"I'm not myself since Dad died.

"Oh, Mom."

We hold each other, both feeling the pain and the loss. We cry aloud together. I understand. I would be lost without Dick. Mom is much too needy to live alone.

"Mom, remember, before Dad died, he said not to make any major decisions for a year. Well, it has been over a year. You followed his wishes. Why don't you come and live with us now?" After I say it, I close my eyes as if expecting some reverberations. I wonder how Mom would feel leaving her place of birth, childhood, and retirement. She has been an officer in the Garden Club and was active in cultural affairs. On the other hand, her brothers and sisters are dead. She has only one family member left in town. All of her immediate family members are up North or out West. Then, again, she has lived in Chicago before and the area is familiar to her. I hold my breath waiting for her answer.

"I think it would be best."

I am overcome with relief. I can't picture myself going back up North and leaving Mom by herself. I call my brother, Sonny, to see what he thinks about Mom moving in with us. He lives on the West Coast. I tell him about the unpaid bills and her forgetfulness. He suggests that Mom be placed in a nursing home in her small town. I am appalled. I say, "How often would you come to see her?" He says, "Two times a year is the most I can manage. I have a job, you know."

I slam down the phone. I get the feeling that I am expected to do all of the care-giving. I sense that he will be available to accept or reject, to analyze, or to evaluate my recommendations. He will not be available for anything else. That feeling proved to be right. I don't have the heart to tell Mom what her son recommended. She doesn't need a nursing home at this time. Maybe someday, it will be necessary, but not now. Besides, I want her to come and live with us. We have one senior citizen living with us and it is okay.

We hug again. This time, we hug and laugh and hug and laugh. Then, we get serious. There are things to do…a house to sell…packing to be done.

4

Fast Friends

Love's stricken "why"
Is all that love can speak-
Built of but just a syllable
The hugest hearts that break.

—Emily Dickinson, 1876

The house sells right away because it is priced below market value. Mom gives the buyers most of her furniture. That leaves her bedroom set, pictures, and clothes to be transported to Illinois. Moving day goes very smoothly, thanks to help from Louvenia. The moving company packs all of Mom's things which she has not given away.

Louvenia escorts Mom to the plane bound for Chicago. She has senior citizen services and gets lots of attention. We meet the plane in Chicago. We are relieved that everything has worked smoothly and are also happy to have Mom come to our home. She is all smiles. I feel that she is also greatly relieved. We drive home and explain that we have arranged her bedroom temporarily until her moving van arrives. When her furniture arrives in the van, she can arrange her own bedroom set with our help.

The day comes when the moving van arrives from Georgia. I am surprised when Mom's ten-year old car is driven out of the van. The insurance isn't paid. Mom doesn't have an Illinois driver's license or plate, and the cost to move the car far exceeds its value.

Within a few days, Mom is happily settled in her own bedroom with her own furniture and clothes and belongings. Helen, Dick's mother, is thrilled to have company during the day. Mom's room is upstairs and Helen's room is downstairs. Helen could not manage the stairs. We converted our family room into her bedroom complete with her own furniture and belongings. Each has her own space.

They have a few weeks of adjustment and bickering. Then things settle down and Mom and Helen become fast friends. We call them Mutt and Jeff because Helen is very tall and Mom is short. Helen has lived with us for many years because she is no longer able to live alone. She can't see to cook or read, but she can watch television if she sits a few feet from the set. Her pacemaker seems to be working fine. She has occasional bouts of diarrhea and nausea due to cancer. She was born in Sweden and has very definite opinions. We fondly remember the days when she would make her delicious cardamom coffee cakes and scrumptious Swedish pancakes. Those days, however, are over. Helen has a matter-of-fact way and is very practical and seldom shows affection. Mom, on the other hand, is very affectionate and a dreamer, not very practical at times. Together, they share the best of each. Helen has become more affectionate and Mom has become more practical. A loving home can work wonders.

They spend most of their days talking about the past until Helen's television program comes on. Then Mom reads. I pack them a lunch like those they used to pack for us as children. In the late afternoon, Dick, Jeff, and I come home from work and talk and laugh and eat and feel content. Some of our friends called us saints for taking them in. They don't think about the many years when these ladies took care of us. Besides, adding love in a home expands the love. We have a circle of love, but we are definitely not saints!

One day, Mom starts talking about her need to visit her birthplace one more time. She becomes obsessed with the idea. We don't want her to have any regrets so we work out arrangements for her to fly with senior citizen services. We take her to the airport and help her with boarding. The stewardess assures us that she will watch over Mom. Mom's nephew from Macon will meet her plane and take her to her hometown. She will spend two weeks visiting friends and her cousin.

Unfortunately, Helen becomes ill a few days before Mom is to leave. Mom is hesitant to go, but decides that so many arrangements have been made for her benefit that she decides to go ahead. Helen becomes progressively sicker and Dick finally persuades her to go to the doctor. She walks into the doctor's office and sits for a few minutes before the nurse motions for her to come to the examining room. She walks to the examining bed, lies down, and passes out. The Doctor calls the ambulance service and she is taken to the hospital. As Helen is dying, her first great grandchild, Ryan, is born. I have often heard that when somebody dies, a baby is born. What a beautiful thought.

Helen's body is riddled with cancer. She has lived with us for eight years and we will miss her. Our grief is shared by our friends and family. Our daughter, Laurie, is trying to perfect her Grandmother's cardamom coffee cake. Both of her grandsons and her granddaughter make Swedish pancakes. Helen lives on in our hearts and bellies with her recipes.

Mom returns after Helen's death and funeral and she is distraught over the loss of Helen. She is saddened by not being able to say "Goodbye" again to a loved one. Mom seems to feel a lack of closure again and seemed stressed. The unraveling continues. She is happy, though, with her first great-grandchild.

5

To Drive or Not To Drive

I felt a Cleaving in my Mind-
As if my Brain had split-
I tried to match it-Seam by Seam-
But could not make them fit.

The thought behind, I strove to join
Unto the thought before-
But Sequence ravelled out of Sound
Like Balls-upon a floor.

—Emily Dickinson, 1864

Mom's old Chevy has been parked on the side of the house ever since the moving van left. One day, Mom asks for help in getting her Illinois driver's license. She is physically fit and alert most of the time so I agree to help her study the driver's manual. We work for two weeks. On days when she is confused, we put it away. On days when she is alert, we make progress.

I start out with oral questioning and later, write a test for her to fill out. We practice driving around our suburban village during the middle of the day when there is less traffic. Mom is feeling confident that she can pass the test. She is adamant that I take her soon.

Mom wakes up early on a Saturday morning and seems especially alert. I think, "Now or never." The weather is clear and cool. The sun is shining. I can see no obstacles. Mom is excited and wants me to quiz her on the way to the driver's license facility. She answers most of the questions. After we park, I go over the street signs with her. She knows them all. She is an intelligent person and I am proud of her persistence and determination. Helping her to drive again is one of the few things she has asked of me after moving in with us. In the deep recesses of my heart, I wonder how long she will be able to drive as well as how long she should drive. I turn off the ignition. Mom runs around to my side of the car and hugs me.

"You're wonderful for helping me. You'll get your reward someday."

"Mom, I'm happy to help you."

"You're a beautiful person."

"Thanks, Mom. Let's go do it."

"Do it."

We wait in line for a half-hour to get the forms. Then, we take a number and wait another forty-five minutes. Mom chats about her grandchildren and comments with the people around her. She seems lighthearted.

Then her number is called. She is given a test of several pages and told to go to a special area to complete the test. I watch her as she works on the pages. She doesn't look up once but keeps focused on the papers. When she is finished, she walks up to the desk and hands the lady her papers. The lady quickly checks her answers. She has passed on the written test with an above average score. She fails to remember, however, two of the street signs on the second part. To pass, one has to get 100% on the street signs, so she has failed the test. Her eyes well up with tears. The lady says, "You can take it again."

"Sister, I'm sorry. I forgot."

"That's okay. You can take it again."

"May I take it now?"

"Let's go across the street to the coffee shop and go over the street signs. I'll buy lunch."

"That sounds good, honey. You're so good to me."

Mom is always complimenting me. She is my biggest fan. But, then, she usually finds positive things to say to and about other people too. She is upbeat and smiling most of the time. People love being around her. Coupled with her sense of humor and affectionate touches, she is one special person.

Lunch is spent with stop signs and other highway markers.

"Okay, Sister, I'm ready." Recently, I notice that Mom reverts to calling me Sister when she is stressed. I'm sure the retesting is stressful. It would be for me.

She goes up to the counter for the second time, gets her papers, finishes them and turns them in. She passed! Her eyes twinkle. Her grin is pure gloat.

"I passed. I passed."

"Yea, Mom"

This joy brings back memories when my children passed their driving tests. It signaled independence for them. We hug and Mom takes another number. She has to pass the driving test now. I notice as we wait this time that she is wringing her hands and is moving around a lot in her chair. Finally, her number is called. A tall, portly gentleman approaches her and says, "Let's go. Where's your car?"

Mom looks at me and says, "C'mon Sister."

"I'm sorry, Ma'am. No passengers allowed."

Mom looks crestfallen and leads the man to her car. She evidently thought that I could go with her. She has not driven alone since leaving her Southern home. I stand at the window watching her. She starts the car and heads, with jumps and starts, toward a busy street. There is a stop sign before entering the street. Mom not only doesn't stop, but she accelerates as she turns the corner into ongoing traffic. Her turn signal isn't on either. The sound of screeching brakes and horns follow as two cars approaching her on the busy street avoid hitting her. My heart is pounding. Mom drives on down the street and out of sight.

Within a few minutes, the loud speaker bellows, "Will Jennie Swanson please come to the front desk?" I am met by Mom and a visibly shaken man who is sweating profusely.

"She should not be on the streets. She's an accident waiting to happen. It's not safe," he says with urgency.

"Okay, thank you, Sir." I look at Mom.

"I'm sorry, Sister. I just couldn't do it."

"It's Okay, Mom. We'll drive you wherever you want to go. You don't need a license when you have a chauffeur." I realize that this is the beginning of the loss of independence for Mom.

"You did a good job on the written test, Mom." She is quiet on the drive home. Then she says, "At least I tried." I remembered her words to me as a child, "Don't say, 'I can't.' Say, 'I will try'".

6

Paranoia Sets In

Fairer though Fading-as the day
Into the Darkness dips away-
Half her Complexion of the Sun-
Hindering-Haunting-Perishing-

Rallies Her Glow, like a dying Friend-
Teasing with glittering Amend-
Only to aggravate the Dark
Through an expiring-perfect-look-

—Emily Dickinson, 1864

Mom generally sleeps through the night. She rarely naps during the day. She is beginning to spend more time looking out the window and less time reading, her favorite pastime. We give her some music and books on tape to entertain her somewhat.

She is clearly having trouble with time concepts. She asks, "What time is it?" over and over. We buy her a watch with large numerals. This helps for a time. Then she keeps misplacing the watch. She asks if we are going to have lunch soon. In reality, lunch was over just a short time ago. At these times, she has no idea what day it is, and certainly, no idea of the month or year. One day, Mom approaches me.

"Someone took my money."

"Where was your money?"

"It was in my purse."

"Let's go look. Nobody would take your money. There are only Dick, and Jeff and I and we wouldn't take your money."

"I said someone took my money, my five dollar bill." Her face becomes strained. She glares at me.

"It's that boy who lives next door to me."

"What boy, Mom?"

I realize that Mom is talking about Jeff. She doesn't remember his name. He is her grandson and she doesn't even recognize him. I am shocked. I know that Jeff would never take her money. We search her room and find her money under her pillow.

This is the first of many episodes of her increasing paranoia. She talks about a neighbor who takes her out to lunch. Mom says she does it because Mom pays, when actually, the neighbor paid. She says the neighbor pumps her for personal information about the family. Knowing the neighbor well, I doubt the accusations.

Mom has been hiding more things and doesn't remember the hiding places. We learn to listen to her complaints, search with her, and try to distract her if the items cannot be found. We learn that it is futile to disagree with her. It only upsets her more.

It is difficult to deal with the paranoia, because we don't know what's causing it. We also don't know that paranoia is often present in Alzheimer's disease. Our family operates on trust and her frequent suspicions about money missing or something being taken is disquieting. Mom is becoming, at times, someone I don't know.

We usually find whatever is missing in the strangest places (in the refrigerator, plants, toilet, etc.). Much later, we begin to realize that some of our things are missing. We laugh and say, "It runs in the family." As time goes on, we stop laughing. I go to my dresser to get underpants and find the drawer empty. They show up later in a hiding place, always in her room. One day, she takes my appointment book. I am frantic until I find it between the mattress and the box springs of Mom's bed.

About the same time, Mom occasionally has difficulty finding a word to express her thoughts. She uses an inappropriate word in a sentence. She knows it is not correct and says, "I think I'm losing my mind." I fear that she might be right. My denial is beginning to weaken.

During this time, Dick and I experience many conflicting feelings. We are sad because Mom has always been so loving and kind. Now, we are seeing a strange and sinister look in her eyes when she is accusatory. We are feeling frustrated because she is constantly taking our things. We are angry because we hate the chaos this is creating in our lives.

We decide we have to do something. Dick puts key locks on our bedroom door and on Jeff's door. We learn to count to 10 before responding to accusations. Then, we remind ourselves to respond with loving words. This is a challenge because it's so annoying. We start using relaxation techniques with Mom. I remember how effective they are with preschoolers. We talk softly if she is upset. We hug her frequently and rub, not pat, her back. She loves this. I fix her a cup of warm Ovaltine. Initially, we gave her a glass of wine before dinner, but the wine made her groggy and unsteady on her feet.

I often sit next to her and put my arm around her as we talk. It's just like my days as a nursery school teacher. All of these things seem to help, especially the touching. I think older, single people may be touch-deprived.

Mom's memory for past events is good but she is slowly becoming unable to recall recent events. Because of the memory loss, the paranoia, and the word-finding problems, we decide to take Mom for a checkup by her doctor.

7

The Doctor's Appointment

God made no act without a cause,
Nor heart without an aim,
Our inference is premature,
Our premises to blame.

—Emily Dickinson, 1870

The doctor's appointment is at 10 A.M. This means we have to get up at 7 A.M. The doctor's office is only fifteen minutes away, but getting Mom up, showered, dressed and fed is a major production.

I go to her bed and hold her small, bony hand covered with age spots.

"Wake up, Mom. We're going to see Dr. Sivad today."

"That's okay. I feel fine. I don't need to see a doctor."

"I'm glad you feel fine. Let's go brag about it to Dr. Sivad."

"Oh, okay."

Mom sits up quickly on the side of the bed. Except for a few paranoid episodes, some speech and memory problems, and difficulty dressing and bathing independently, Mom is still the sweet, caring person she always was. She has a sense of humor and loves to laugh. As she sits on the bed, I can see that she is confused about what to do.

"Mom, the shower water is just right. Are you ready?"

"I'm coming, darling."

I help her take off her nightgown and invite her to step into the shower. She stands under the steady stream of water, not moving. I hand her the washcloth with soap on it.

"Mom, please wash your arms."

"Good, now wash your chest."

Each time I rinse out the washcloth and put soap on it, I have to invite her to wash another part of her body; otherwise, she would just stand there. It seems to take forever. She needs so many invitations. I call them invitations to remind myself not to demand and to be patient. It's a way of respecting her dignity. It reminds me of the many invitations I have given in the past to children in a pre-school special education program. It was important to help them maintain their self-image and learn at the same time. There are times when I grit my teeth and "invite" Mom too loudly or too firmly. I never gritted my teeth like this as a teacher, but I wasn't on 24 hour duty then. The frustration is usually my own fault because I have not given Mom enough "idling" time which she seems to need. I wash her back and she soaps her hair with shampoo.

"Okay, now, lean forward."

"Good. Now, step back."

"Okay, now hold your head up."

"Good job. Now, you are all finished." Praising good behavior was also a part of preschool teaching.

Mom steps out of the shower and complains about being cold. She just stands there and shivers. She has no inkling how to solve this problem. I quickly cover her with a towel and wipe her dry. She does not seem to be able to dry herself except for her arms and stomach.

As I dress her, she talks nonstop. She is a positive and loving person and greets each day with enthusiasm.

"What a beautiful day."

"You're so pretty. I love you." And on she goes.

She walks down the stairs and goes to the breakfast table and sits down. She's like a queen in some ways. I draw her bath or shower, put out her clothes and, now, she waits for breakfast to be served. Maybe not like a queen, but a young child. I try to give her choices, an important part of a young child's experience.

"Would you like waffles or cereal?"

"I'll have cereal, please."

"Oatmeal or corn flakes?"

"Oatmeal, please."

Mom went to charm school as a young Southern belle. Her manners have always been impeccable.

While Mom is eating, I run upstairs to shower and dress. When I come down, Mom is sitting and looking out the window. The oatmeal is untouched.

"How about taking a bite?"

"Okay."

With constant invitations, Mom finally finishes her oatmeal. I help her with her coat. Then, she wanders upstairs while I go to get my coat.

There is silence.

"Mom, it is time to go."

I have the feeling that I am about to "lose it" so I sit down and take a couple of sips of coffee and try to decelerate. I wish I had time for a short meditation. It would calm me down. I'm finding myself more on edge lately. My job is very challenging and time consuming and taking care of Mom leaves me precious little time for much else. I feel the need for some respite care for myself. When I go upstairs, Mom is undressing.

"What are you doing?" I shout.

"It's time for bed."

"No, it's not. C'mon Mom. We're going out." At this point, I feel like going into another room and letting out a loud scream but it would scare Mom to death. I dress her quickly with no invitations this time and off we go.

I always grumble when people see her and say she looks fine and there doesn't look like there's anything wrong with her. Sure, she looks fine because I take care of her. If she had to dress herself, she might put the arms of the sweater on her legs (which she has done many times), or put on a bra backwards, if at all, and forget to comb her hair. She might also put on four blouses.

Many other people who care for the elderly tell me that casual observers often question the validity of an assessment of a person's problems when the person can make "small talk" and smile and especially when they look presentable. This is true with Mom. When I share my frustrations and concerns with some friends, they say, "She looks fine to me," or "At least, she's a lovable person." You would have to live twenty-four hours with her to understand the type of care that she requires. A superficial view does not reveal the reality of the problems. I have an expanded appreciation of parents of severely handicapped children who often said, "You have to live with them to know what it's like." You would have to walk in their shoes. You would have to walk in my shoes.

As Mom sits in the doctor's waiting room, she looks like a sweet little old lady, smiling in response to others, saying hello to children, and in general, looking very appropriate. She has times like these. As we wait for the doctor in the examining room, Mom becomes anxious. She says, "Let's go," several times. After thirty minutes, the doctor opens the door briskly and says, "Hello, Cleo. How are you?"

"I'm fine."

"What seems to be the problem?"

"I don't have any problems. I feel fine."

I join in. "Doctor, Mom seems to be in good physical condition but she worries about her mind. She's forgetful and suspicious about others. Every once in a while, she'll say, I think I'm losing my mind."

"How old are you, Cleo?" he asks.

"Jennie, how old am I?" She looks pleadingly at me.

I tell the doctor.

What year is it?" he continues.

"Tell him, Sister."

This pattern continues with each question. I tell Doctor Sivad that she does not know the answer to any of the questions. Then, I take a deep breath and ask, "Doctor, does Mom have Alzheimer's disease?"

"No, she's fine. We all forget things as we grow older. We'll take some blood tests to rule out the problems. We'll get back to you in a few days with the results." As we walk out of the office, I think, "He's nuts. Something is definitely wrong."

A week later, the nurse from the doctor's office calls to say that Mom's blood tests are fine. No further tests are needed. I had such hopes for help when I walked into that office. What can I do? Where can I turn? I have to do something.

8

Finding Answers

Were it to be the last
How infinite would be
What we did not suspect was marked-
Our final interview.

—Emily Dickinson, 1870 (?)

I decide to trust my instincts and my education. I know that something is definitely wrong with Mom. Her symptoms can't just be explained away as normal aging. Damn that doctor! In my gut, I know that she has Alzheimer's disease.

I had worked for eight years in a major medical center. One thing I had learned was that medicine is not a precise science. I was also aware that doctors are often uncomfortable with illnesses where there is no treatment or cure. Alzheimer's disease is one of those. It's difficult to diagnose in the early stage. Other conditions have similar symptoms. The definitive diagnosis may be made only through an autopsy, the examination of brain tissue after death. Other tests may be given to the living patient to rule out other illnesses which can be treated such as depression, adverse drug reactions, head injuries, stroke, and others. After other illnesses are ruled out, observing the patient over time lends weight to the probable diagnosis of Alzheimer's disease if the symptoms remain and gradually get worse. The diagnosis is more evident if the patient is in a more advanced stage of the illness. At least, Mom's doctor could have referred me to a specialist for consultation after hearing our concerns.

My grown children are asking questions about their grandma. I decide to research the current literature on Alzheimer's disease. As I drive to the library through the back roads of my village, my thoughts pop up like fireworks on a fourth of July evening. "What is it?" "Why Mom?" "What am I going to do?" "What about my job?" "Can I handle this?" "What will it cost?" Mostly, I think about Mom. "What must she be thinking?" "How does it feel to lose your 'now'?" "Is she scared?" "What help does she need?" "What can we do together to make things easier for her?"

Tears flow down my cheeks as I imagine what it must be like to be unable to think of familiar words, to be unable to dress myself, to be unable to bathe independently, to be unable to cook, and to be unable to remember what just had happened. I would be terrified.

The library is filled with school children because it is Saturday. They are reading, chatting, laughing, and some are studying. The place is alive with life. It's a good place for me today. It's a reminder that life goes on.

I look up Alzheimer's disease. Yes, I know that AD (Alzheimer's disease) is a progressive and degenerative disease and it attacks the brain and affects behavior, thinking, and memory. It is the most common form of dementia. The disease was first described by Alois Alzheimer in 1907. I didn't know that AD is the fourth leading cause of death in adults. I realize that I am not alone. There must be many people like me struggling to understand and to survive this life challenge.

I scan the stacks of books to find something about the symptoms. It seems that symptoms may include gradual memory loss, impairment of judgment, gradual decline in performance of routine tasks, confusion or disorientation, paranoia, personality changes, and language and learning difficulties. Mom has all of these.

As I sit in the library, the recognition, the confirmation gradually absorbs me. My denial is slowly stripped away. I guess I knew it all along but I didn't want to face the brutal truth. I read voraciously through parts of selected texts. I scan others. Finally, exhausted, I gather up 15 books to take home. I am like Mom in one way. This is going to be my challenge. I accept that Mom has Alzheimer's disease. Although I know it in my gut, I will have the diagnosis confirmed by a medical doctor. Mom deserves that and, besides, other conditions/illnesses can cause Alzheimer's symptoms. We need to rule those out.

I do think that, in the future, the diagnosis will be made by teams consisting of doctors, nurse specialists, developmental specialists (like myself), radiologists, psychologists, and neuropsychologists. Once other medical conditions are ruled out, behavioral symptoms must be observed and evaluated over time. Some major medical centers and some hospitals use such teams now. Some doctors refer patients to them. I wish Mom's doctor had referred her to a team in Chicago.

When I arrive home, Dick and Mom are sitting at the table chatting over a cup of coffee. I sit down and share my findings with them. My family has never been one to keep secrets from each other. I put everything out on the table. Mom and Dick listen intently. Mom is having a good day and seems very alert. After a few minutes of silence and a prayer, Mom says she has known for some time that she has Alzheimer's disease. Her greatest fear is not the disease but how it affects us. She says she is glad it is out in the open.

"Mom, we're a family. We're in this together."

"Maybe I should go to a nursing home. I don't want to be a burden." This statement is made several years after Mom's son (my brother) recommended a nursing home.

"This is your home. We'll take care of you as long as we can." I add the last part quickly. Dick nods his head and takes Mom's hand and squeezes it. I am careful not to promise that we will never consider a nursing home. I had just read several accounts of people promising this, only to feel tremendous guilt when a nursing home becomes the best of poor alternatives.

"Mom, does it scare you when you forget something?" Dick asks.

"Yes, but mostly, I'm embarrassed."

We sit for hours drinking wine, comforting Mom, hugging, and asking her advice about what helps. She does a lot of reminiscing about her life. She gives a life interview, as some call it. I wish I had her comments on tape. Mom says she is well satisfied with her life and has been very happy for the most part. She seemed relieved and very sleepy as we finish off some cheesecake. She mentions a regret. She has never gone to Hawaii. We make plans to go. Mom has only a few sips of wine but when she stands, her legs are wobbly. Dick and Mom and I all agree. No more wine.

Dick picks her up like an infant and carries her upstairs and gently puts her down on the bed. She looks so peaceful. I don't remove her sweat suit. I just take off her shoes and socks, cover her up, and kiss her good night. It reminds me of the times I used to put my children to bed. This time, there is no bedtime story. Mom is fast asleep.

Then, Dick and I talk until late into the night. Dick says, "I don't want to die like your Mom. It's like she's dying with her eyes open, and slowly, at that. I want to die quickly and at home. I want to go feet first out of this house."

I talk about how relieved I am that Mom acknowledges that she has Alzheimer's disease and that he supports me in taking care of Mom. I don't want our children to be faced with my care in my old age. I think we should get long-term care insurance. We ramble on and make plans for Hawaii. We'll both go with her, of course. Thank goodness, we can afford to go. We don't want Mom to have any regrets. Thank goodness for Dick. I don't know how people handle this alone.

9

More Questions, More Answers

This is a Blossom of the Brain-
A small-italic Seed
Lodged by Design or Happening
The Spirit fructified-

Shy as the Wind of his Chambers
Swift as a Freshet's Tongue
So of the Flower of the Soul
Its process is unknown.

When it is found, a few rejoice
The Wise convey it Home
Carefully cherishing the spot
If other Flower become.

When it is lost, that Day shall be
The Funeral of God,
Upon his Breast, a closing Soul
The Flower of our Lord.

—Emily Dickinson, 1864

I search for answers to questions about Alzheimer's disease.

What is Alzheimer's disease?

Alzheimer's disease is the most common form of dementia. Dementia is not a disease but a set of symptoms that accompanies certain conditions or diseases. Alzheimer's is one of the diseases of dementia. Others include Parkinson's disease, Huntington's disease, multi-infarct dementia, Creutzfeldt-Jacob disease, Pick's disease, and Lewy body dementia.

According to the Alzheimer's Association, Alzheimer's disease is:

> Not a normal part of aging
> Not covered by most private health insurance
> Not limited to the elderly
> Not currently curable, but help is available

Alzheimer's is a progressive, degenerative disease that attacks the brain and results in impaired memory, thinking, and behavior. It is the fourth leading cause of death in adults and affects men and women almost equally.

What causes Alzheimer's disease?

The cause or causes are not known. Some areas being researched include genetic disposition, a slow virus, environmental toxins, free radicals, an inflammation, the AADL (amyloid-derived diffusible ligand) protein, and immunological changes. It appears that Alzheimer's develops because of a complex series of events over time.

What does it cost to care for an Alzheimer's patient?

According to the Alzheimer's Association:

> U.S. society spends at least $100 billion a year on AD. Neither Medicare nor most private health insurance covers the long term care most patients need. More than 7 out of 10 people with Alzheimer's disease live at home. Almost 75% of the home care is provided by family and friends. The remainder is "paid" care costing an average of $12,500 per year. Families pay almost all of that out-of-pocket.
>
> Alzheimer's disease is the third most expensive disease in the United States after heart disease and cancer.

According to the Met Life Survey of Nursing Homes and Home Care Costs (Executive Summary, Sept. 2004):

> The average daily rate for a private room in a nursing home is $192 or $70,080 annually. The average daily rate for a semiprivate room in a nursing home is $169 or $61,685 annually.

What percentages of patients in nursing homes have Alzheimer's disease?

More than 50% of all nursing home patients suffer from Alzheimer's disease or a related disorder.

Who gets Alzheimer's disease?

The most important risk factor for Alzheimer's disease is age. According to ADEAR (Alzheimer's Disease Education and Referral), four million people have the disease in the U.S. Three percent are age 65-74. Nearly half of those over 85 have the disease.

Is help available?

The National Alzheimer's Association (1-800-272-3900 & web site www.alz.org) provides information on sources of help, respite care, educational seminars, books and pamphlets, research, support and self-help groups, fund-raising, referral, and "someone to stand by you." Local chapters may be of special help and may be accessed through the National Alzheimer's Organization in Chicago.

The Department of Aging (800-677-1116) has resources for help. Local offices can inform you of local services. Other caregiver sources are Children of Aging Parents (215-945-6900) and the Eldercare Hotline (800-677-1116) and the American Association of Retired Persons (AARP) at www.aarp.org/life/caregiving. The Alzheimer's Disease and Referral Center of the National Institute on Aging may be reached at 800-438-4380 or at www.alzheimers.org.

Newspapers often list the meeting place and times of support/self-help groups. Nursing homes, hospitals, universities, and junior colleges will occasionally offer seminars. Other resources include home health agencies, hospital social workers, veteran's administration, elder legal services, geriatric care managers, adult day care programs, mental health clinics, religious counselors, private therapists, family service agencies, and religious institutions.

Reading about Alzheimer's disease may be helpful. For children, there is Maria Shriver's book, *What's Happening to Grandpa*. For practical advice for caregivers, *The 36 Hour Day: A Family Guide to Caring For Persons with Alzheimer's Illnesses. Memory Loss in Later Life* by Nancy L. Mace and Peter V. Robins is also a valuable resource. *Living in the Labyrinth* by Diana Friel McGowin describes the author's own experience with AD. The book, *Mayo Clinic on Alzheimer's Disease,* edited by Ronald Petersen, Ph.D., includes diagrams and photographs to demonstrate the brain impact of AD as well as an in-depth treatise on understanding the disease, treatment, and care giving. *Preventing Alzheimer's* by William Rodman Shankle, M.S., M.D. and Daniel G. Amen, M.D. describes ways to help prevent, detect and halt AD. The PBS Home Video of *The Forgetting* based on the book by David Shenk gives a visual side of AD.

I know that my family and friends will be my best support. At any rate, no one is alone in this journey. There is help out there.

When is Alzheimer's disease usually diagnosed?

Most people are given the probable diagnosis in their 60's, 70's, or 80's. An increasing number are being identified in their 40's and 50's. These are referred to as Early-onset AD. I mention probable diagnosis because a definitive diagnosis cannot be made except by an autopsy after death.

Is screening available?

No generally accepted screening is available. There are an increasing number of physicians who specialize in geriatric care and Alzheimer's. A simple questionnaire given to a patient may provide some insight and be the basis for additional testing and/or referral. Genetic screening is available but the function of genetic knowledge in Alzheimer's disease needs more study. Screening should be approached with caution until further studies with larger populations are completed. As more effective medications are developed for the early stage, screening may be helpful. *Preventing Alzheimer's* by William Rodman Shackle and Daniel G. Amen (G.P.Putnam's Sons, N.Y., 2004) provides current information about screening.

Is Alzheimer's genetic?

According to Medline Plus, we know the three major genes for Early-onset Alzheimer's and one gene for Late-onset AD.

A major role in AD is played by a gene called apolipoprotein E or apoE. This gene may protect some people from developing the disease, while a flawed form of the gene increases the risk significantly. Each cell in the body has two copies of the apoE gene which is on chromosome 19. People with two copies of the apoE4 gene have 11-17 times greater risk of developing AD. Even with one apoE gene, the risk is five times greater than among people with no apoE4 genes (Roses et al, 1993). Roses of Duke University reported that 90% of the people with two apoE4 genes will have A.D. by age 80. Some say that E4 is a risk factor and not a cause. More studies are needed.

How many Americans have Alzheimer's disease?

The National Institute on Aging estimates that four million Americans have the disease. Nineteen million Americans say their families have been touched by the disease. It is estimated that 14 million people will have the disease by 2050 unless a cure is found.

How long does a person have the disease?

From the onset of symptoms, a person may live from three to twenty years or more. The average is ten years. This information is not too helpful. It seems that a person can have memory with a lack of further deterioration for three years and still be in the early stages of AD. Once the person starts to decline, the decline seems to continue at the same rate. It seems that the rate of decline can be estimated and is quite stable for each individual. The rate is determined after mental abilities, other than memory, begin to decline. This information was found in a study by Haxby et al, 1992. In addition, the study reported that the fastest rates of decline were four times faster than the slowest rates of decline. Clearly, more information is needed to determine the basis for predicting the length of the illness. New medications are on the market which claim to delay some symptoms.

Can the onset of the disease be delayed?

David Snowdon, University of Kentucky, has been studying nuns for several years. The nuns do not seem to suffer from dementia, Alzheimer's, and other degenerative diseases as early or as severely as the general population. He found that those who earn college degrees, who teach, who constantly challenge their minds, live longer than those nuns who cleaned rooms or worked in the kitchen.

Snowdon believes, with surplus brain branching and connections, messages can be rerouted. As a former teacher, I know that bored students may be fodder for behavior problems. I say, "Keep them productively occupied." It looks as if productive activity in old age is important too. I know that bored students can be "rerouted." What about AD patients?

More recently, Snowdon has found a strong link between the nuns' youthful writing skills and their late-life risk for developing brain lesions and Alzheimer's disease. It appears that those with high linguistic ability may have a brain which is resistant to AD, while those with low linguistic ability in young adulthood may be already manifesting the disease. This study suggests that Alzheimer's may be a lifelong disease process.

Snowdon also found that "Over 95% of people will develop the protein deposits, the so-called plaque and tangle lesions of Alzheimer's if they live to be old enough. Yet most will somehow escape showing any significant symptoms of this disease." This is a new area for research.

Other current findings by researchers strengthen the cholesterol and Alzheimer's link. This study was reported in the January, 2004 issue of the *Archives of Neurology*. The study links cholesterol-lowering drugs called statins with a reduced risk of AD.

Other studies have suggested that a range of things may reduce the risk of developing Alzheimer's, including weight, diet, nutrition, normal blood pressure levels, exercise, and cholesterol levels. More study is needed.

A new medication is now available for late stage Alzheimer's as well as the early stage. The drug targets a neurotransmitter called glutamate that appears, in large quantities, to damage cells. Improvement has been seen in some patients in memory, behavior, and everyday living skills. It is not known how much time AD is delayed by the medication. It might be two to three years.

The book previously mentioned, *Preventing Alzheimer's,* includes specific suggestions for preventing, delaying, and even halting the disease.

Do anti-inflammatory drugs help?

Dr. John Breiter, Duke University, studied 50 sets of elderly and non-identical twins. He found that twins taking anti-inflammatory drugs were four times less likely to develop AD or to develop it many years later.

Another study by neuroscientist, Joseph Rogers, Director of the Sun Health Research Institute, Sun City, Arizona, gave an anti-inflammatory drug to fourteen Alzheimer's patients and a placebo to fourteen others. Patients given the drug did not get worse and improved slightly. Patients given the placebo continued their mental decline. More and larger studies are needed to confirm these findings.

People with rheumatoid arthritis rarely develop AD. They probably take anti-inflammatory drugs. This helps to support the theory that Alzheimer's may be caused by a destructive inflammatory process in the brain.

It is premature and possibly dangerous, however, for people to start taking aspirin or other anti-inflammatory drugs without medical attention and until further studies are completed.

Is there a memory drug available?

There are some drugs which may improve memory. They must be prescribed by a physician after a careful evaluation.

What are tangles and plaques?

Over time, the disease destroys brain cells leaving behind abnormalities called tangles and plaques. Tangles are dense insoluble clots of material inside damaged brain cells (neurons). Plaques appear on the outside. They are clumps of special protein intertwined with dead and dying branches of surrounding nerves.

Researchers have found beta-amyloid protein (the major component of the neuritic plaques that show the presence of Alzheimer's) in the skin of patients who appear to have AD. Maybe, someday, a simple skin test will reveal the disease.

What brain areas are affected?

The first nerves to die are in the area known as the limbic system which is deep within the brain and controls emotion and memory. As the destruction spreads toward the surface of the brain, language and movement are affected. As the damage further advances, the motor cortex is affected and the person with Alzheimer's is unable to walk, talk, or swallow.

On that note, I decided that it was time to concentrate on Mom's happiness for the time she had left. She is literally dying to live. I knew that I would continue to search for answers about this perplexing disease. Many of these answers will change over time due to new findings in research.

10

The Brain Drain

The Brain, within its Groove
Runs evenly- and true-
But let a Splinter swerve-
'Twere easier for You-

To put a Current back-
When Floods have slit the Hills-
And scooped a Turnpike for Themselves-
And trodden out the Mills-

—Emily Dickinson, 1862

I have an educational background in neuropsychology and I realize that Alzheimer's disease is primarily a disease of the brain. I try to explain the complex workings of the brain to my grandchildren when they ask questions. Why does Great-gramma keep asking questions over and over again? Why doesn't she remember me? Why is she growing backwards instead of forward? We have kept them informed throughout their Great-gramma's decline.

The grandchildren have had a unique learning experience. At first, they were frightened by it because it is called a disease. They thought they might "catch" it. They slowly became comfortable being around her and other elderly people with disabilities. I am touched by my grandchildren's kindnesses. Their empathy is, at times, inspirational. They seem to be able to deal with the situation when they are informed.

I explain to them that the brain is like a giant computer, only it is more complex and can do more things than any computer you can buy today. Scientists are learning more about the brain every day, but it is still a mystery, just as Alzheimer's disease is still a big mystery. No one knows what causes AD or what cures it.

We know that the brain is the master computer of the body functions. It is the central manager or the boss of the body. We know that AD is a disease of the brain. When your master computer (your brain) is mixed up, you're mixed up. Over time you become more mixed up, because your brain is not working right and the communication system in the brain (the connections between the cells) is breaking down.

We make a model of the brain out of clay, and show the grandchildren the two hemispheres and the pathway between them and how Alzheimer's begins deep within the brain.

We can put dots on a blank page and take turns connecting them. We can think of the dots as brain cells and the lines between the dots as connections. This will give them a primitive idea of brain cell structure. I explain that special substances are needed to make the connections work. These substances are called neurotransmitters. There are other structures present on the cells. With AD, some of the dots or cells are missing or dying and the lines are tangled. It is helpful to show a picture of normal brain tissue to compare with the tangles and plaques of AD.

My message to the grandchildren is that Great-gramma cannot help the way she is. Her brain is different and will continue to be different. She would certainly remember them if she could. Depending on the child's understanding, I might stop here with explanations. I would continue and draw pictures if the interest is still present.

Alzheimer's disease ravages the complex brain, not all at once, but slowly over time like grains of sand drifting one by one relentlessly in an egg timer. Autopsies of Alzheimer's patients have shown the loss at the cellular level. Cells are fewer in number and are frequently abnormal. Cell death is the major culprit. Alzheimer's is a disease of disconnection. This is true in more ways than one.

The brain is a new frontier for research. We have yet to unlock its many mysteries, but the brain sciences (neurology, neuropsychology, neurophysiology, neuropharmacology, and others) are rapidly gaining new understandings augmented by new technology (CT scans, MRI, PET, and SPECT analysis and others). Cognitive development has become a bridge between medicine, particularly for the neurosciences, and education.

Memory depends on stimulation. Stimulation is an important factor for the aging population. It now appears that biological changes occur when the brain learns a specific task. Through inactivity, mental functions can be lost. This has implications for caregivers, adult day care, and nursing home staff. "Use it or lose it," as the saying goes. The Alzheimer's patient will lose it anyway, but perhaps the rate may be affected.

While stimulation is important, relaxation is equally important. It is the body's recuperation time. Lack of relaxation and sleep can cause agitation and mood swings in some Alzheimer's patients. I notice a direct correlation between the amount of Mom's night wandering with her general mood and level of agitation during the day.

What can we do to help? We can enjoy our loved one's "now." We can have our loved one evaluated by a research team to add to their data and understanding. We can do fund-raising for research. We can support organizations that contribute to research. We can make sure that our loved one has signed a Living Will and a Durable Power of Attorney while he/she is still competent to do so.

We can make arrangements now for a brain autopsy after death at a medical center doing research on Alzheimer's. A complete autopsy is not necessary. Only brain tissue is needed. Check to make sure if there are any costs. This autopsy will be your loved one's unique contribution. Reading the results may give you additional information. It is often too late to make specific arrangements for an autopsy for research purposes as you sit at the bedside of a dying person. Mom wanted a brain autopsy of her brain. She felt gratified that she could be of help.

Finally, we can take care of ourselves. We can join a support group. We can get respite care. Sometimes we have to schedule time to live our lives too.

The mind is a terrible thing to lose. Ask yourself, "What is the last thing I could do without?" Would it be your functioning brain?

11

The Stages of Alzheimer's Disease

Down Time's quaint Stream
Without an oar
We are enforced to sail
Our Port a secret
Our Perchance a Gale
What Skipper would
Incur the Risk
What Buccaneer would ride
Without a surety from the Wind
Or schedule of the Tide-

—Emily Dickinson

Because of my studies in human growth and development as well as my life experiences, I realize that we are all unique and respond in different ways to different circumstances. I agree with Hans Selye, researcher on stress:

What matters is not so much what happens to us, but the way we take it.

I wonder what is ahead for Mom and me. I wonder how I can prepare for the inevitable decline of Mom's functioning. I can give up or I can or try to meet this challenge. I am aware of her symptoms. Her new doctor and his team have ruled out other illnesses. He says that Mom has "probable Alzheimer's disease." She is on a path leading to death. But, aren't we all!

Where are we going on this path? Dr. Selye also said at a conference that I attended, "The better prepared we are for a stressful event, the better we can handle it." Since I am an education advocate, I return to the library. I find out that there are roughly three stages on this path we are on. Due to denial by the person and the family, the first stage may be subtly absorbed in everyday life and excuses or rationalizations made for behavior. I denied the first stage longer than Mom. She asked me if she had Alzheimer's and I thought the idea was preposterous. Of course, the nun study by Snowdon suggests that Alzheimer's may begin very early in life.

The Initial or First Stage

One of the first signs of Alzheimer's disease is forgetfulness or short-term memory loss. The loss becomes greater over time, sometimes even years before it is recognized as a problem. Stresses such as illness, travel, and change can heighten memory loss. Certainly the sudden deaths of her husband and Helen resulted in a decline of Mom's functioning. Her move to Illinois and her last trip to Georgia probably took their toll.

The person with AD may feel that something is wrong. Mom used to say, "I think I'm losing my mind." She even copied and gave me a poem to help me understand.

> Just a line to say I'm living,
> That I'm not among the dead,
> Tho I'm getting more forgetful,
> And more mixed up in the head.
>
> For sometimes I can't remember,
> When I stand at the foot of the stair,
> If I must go up for something,
> Or if I've just come down from there,
>
> And before the 'fridge so often,
> My poor mind is filled with doubt,
> Have I just put food away, or
> Have I come to take some out?
>
> And there are times when it is dark out,
> With my nightcap on my head,

I don't know if I'm retiring
Or just getting out of bed.

So, if it is time to write you,
There is no need in getting sore,
I may think that I have written,
And don't want to be a bore.

So, remember I do love you,
And wish that you were here,
And now it's nearly mail time,
So I must say, "Goodbye, Dear."

There I stand beside the mailbox
With a face so very red,
Instead of mailing you my letter,
I opened it instead.

—Author Unknown

Even though Mom sensed something was wrong, she coped with the problem by writing reminders to herself. She would cross off each day on the calendar and keep appointments on it. She would carry a small spiral notebook and jot reminders in it. She even wrote notes of encouragement to herself:

For I, the Lord thy God, will hold thy right hand saying unto thee,
Fear not, I will help thee.

Mom wrote a paper titled, "Some Lessons":

If you fail once, get up and try again.
Be ready to help.
A forgiving heart is greater than power.
The way a fellow treats his people shows what he is.

These were some of the ways that Mom met her challenges. She would greet people enthusiastically and affectionately but would say very little, thereby not exposing herself. I remember Dad used to say, "When you're talking, you're not learning." Mom's slant might be, "When you're listening, you're not exposing yourself to ridicule."

Mom knew when she had used an inappropriate word in a sentence and would blush and joke about it. This demeanor kept us from taking the problem seriously for a long time.

As time went on, she had difficulty concentrating and showed flawed judgment like the time she had her 10 year-old car transported to Illinois at a greater cost than its value.

Some people with AD during this stage become depressed. They may appear sad, sleep a lot, lose weight, lose interest in their surroundings and even drink alcohol more than usual. It is important to seek medical attention for depression because treatment may be helpful. Mom didn't appear to be depressed. She was always a positive person who was active and lovable and loving. She did, however, become depressed in a later stage.

Because the symptoms come and go during this stage, the ill person and the family might pin their hopes on the good times and tend to ignore the problem areas as long as they can. The good times give us false hope. This is also a good time to have a medical evaluation. The diagnosis may not be possible during this stage but a checkup provides a baseline for a downward trend of symptoms. Treatment for some symptoms may be possible.

As more supervision of the ill person is needed, the family may begin to openly recognize the problems. The family begins to fill in gaps for the person providing the appropriate word, giving clues for forgetfulness, and providing increasing care.

The Alzheimer's Association provides 10 warning signs:

1. Recent memory loss affects job skills

2. Difficulty performing familiar tasks

3. Problems with language

4. Disorientation of time and place

5. Poor or decreased judgment

6. Problems with abstract thinking

7. Misplacing things

8. Changes in mood or behavior

9. Changes in personality

10. Loss of initiative

Mom exhibited all of these. Some were more troublesome than others.

The Middle Stage

The memory loss becomes more and more severe over time until finally the person no longer recognizes friends and family members. I believe that frequent contact affects memory. Mom recognized only friends and family who were seen frequently. Eventually only a few people are remembered. With Mom, I was the last person she forgot, probably because I was the most consistent person in her life. Finally, no one is recognized. Memory is severely impaired.

Short-term memory is the first to be lost. Mom could not remember what happened recently but she could recall things that happened a long time ago (long-term memory). Eventually, both long and short term memories are lost.

Judgment becomes worse. Mom got to a point where she didn't want to order dinner in a restaurant. She would say, "I'll have whatever you have." Seldom did she ever eat her complete meal. We convinced some restaurants to use the children's menu when ordering for Mom. We tried to give her two choices from which to choose. This worked most of the time. Eventually, she was unable to choose and we simply would order for her.

Social skills become impaired. Mom always told us as children that you don't pass gas in public. But, very often, after a meal in a restaurant, she would walk out and pass gas as she went. Dick and I were initially very embarrassed. As time went on, we would just march single file to the sounds of the "drum roll" as Dick called them.

> Beat! Beat! Drums! Blow! Bugles! Blow!
> Through the windows-through doors-burst like a ruthless force,
> (Exerpt from BEAT! BEAT! DRUMS!)
> Walt Whitman
> *Leaves of Grass*

This was the beginning of our real humanity. We developed an attitude that whatever Mom did was okay. We were not going to be embarrassed by her anymore because our embarrassment punctured her dignity. We were not going to curtail our usual activities with her either. We were going to accept her "as is." Sometimes, we would simply say to others, "It's okay, she has Alzheimer's disease." We should all be so lucky to be accepted "as is". We could simply say, "Its okay, I'm human."

As we shared her AD with others, we found others sharing their experiences with us. Most people had a relative or knew someone with the disease. Their understanding showed us not only that we were not alone, but also the extent of the disease.

Restlessness, wandering, and sleep disturbances also characterize this stage for many. Mom would wander out to our rural mailbox, get the mail, and then, hide it. She would deny doing it. Naturally, she didn't remember. Generally, Mom's wandering was around the house and our yard. She never ventured far. I've heard stories of people with AD wandering off for miles. This would be very difficult to manage.

Mom could sit and stare out the window for hours, then get up and get into all kinds of mischief. Then, she would settle down and stare again. We called it her "revving up time." Later as Dick and I heard Boxcar Willy, a popular Branson, Missouri attraction (prior to his death) sing, "Winds of Yesterday", we thought about Mom's staring differently. Many of the memories in the song would be familiar to Mom. We thought about her mentally going back to earlier days of her life, as in the song, "Winds of Yesterday".

> Sometimes at night when I'm all alone,
> The sounds of the day fade away.
> Alone in my room with my memories,
> The winds of yesterday blow on me.
> I hear the country music on the radio,
> The way it was a long time ago,
> And the sound of Momma's singing
> Comes drifting through the trees,
> When the winds of yesterday blow on me.
>
> I see a moon so bright
> Over cotton fields of white.
> The fragrance of magnolias ride the breeze,
> And that little two-room school
> Where I learned the Golden rule,
> When the winds of yesterday blow on me.
>
> I see children at the ole swimming' hole,
> And fishin' on the river with that ole cane pole
> Each memory is so dear,
> Each face is so clear,
> When the winds of yesterday blow on me.

I can hear the choir sing.
How their voices ring.
I remember the words to each song.
Oh, and that ole preacher man
Once more sets my heart at ease,
When the winds of yesterday blow on me.
When the winds of yesterday blow on me.

Who knows? Mom may have been reliving her wonderful life in Georgia, all within herself, and maybe she was not just staring.

Personality changes started to take place. Most of the time, Mom was her sweet self. Then, suddenly, with no apparent provocation, she would stiffen up and have a sinister look in her eyes. Her pupils were like small penetrating back dots. This look always scared me. It was so unlike Mom. If we didn't do something to soothe her, she would hit or bite. We learned to distract Mom and, often, her mood would quickly change. This is also a good technique for young children. Distraction and soothing words or actions help. Meanwhile, it took us a while to recover from this new behavior of Mom's. It was as if a stranger was living with us at times. The night wandering was a concern for us because our bedrooms were on the second floor. We tied a large rope at the top of the stairs so that she wouldn't fall down. She would wander and forget where her bed was, so she needed someone to guide her back to bed. I did this several times each night. It reminded me of the night feedings when my children were infants.

Mom was unable to calculate, to add or to subtract, but she could still read. It surprised me that many Alzheimer's victims can read during this stage. It is really more of a decoding task than reading because, often, meaning or comprehension is lacking.

The language loss becomes more pronounced with occasional bizarre sentences, having no relevance to the situation and frequently repetitious. At times, there was mumbling. The inability to express thoughts is very frustrating for the person with AD. It is also a serious sign to caregivers as to the mental confusion which is present.

Safety becomes a real issue eventually. We have to be vigilant at times for fear that something terrible might happen. Mom can no longer cook without supervision. We purchased a new cook top with removable knobs which we took off when we were not cooking. We had to keep non-edibles out of the kitchen. Mom would eat anything, even garbage. We put safety caps on the electrical outlets. Appliances were unplugged. We removed all of the unnecessary items from the furniture in her room. These are some of the things one does when making a home safe for toddlers.

Mom tried to eat a dish of fragrant potpourri once. We packed away potentially hazardous materials (matches, medications, cleaning supplies, etc.). We gave away plants which would be poisonous if eaten. She couldn't be trusted not to eat the leaves. We purchased low-heeled, non-skid shoes for her and packed away throw rugs. We used child safety gates to keep her in a three room area while I cooked dinner. She never questioned these gates. Our house is also safer for our grandchildren.

Some AD people cry easily during this stage. Mom didn't. She did occasionally shed tears of happiness. She would frequently ask, "What am I supposed to be doing?" or "Am I okay?" We found that a reassuring, "You're just fine" was all that she needed.

The most difficult symptom for our family, during this stage, was Mom's paranoia. Distrust can undermine a family structure. Until we realized that the paranoia was part of her illness, I had many dark days and nights. My own mother didn't trust me. She was accusing Jeff and Dick of theft.

One night, I was overwhelmed by Mom's paranoia and her care. I was depressed, tired, and felt sorry for myself. I stood up suddenly after dinner and said, "I'm going out."

"Where are you going?" Dick said sensing my sadness and concerned about my apparent urgency to leave.

"Just out."

I got in the car and drove for over an hour. I wept as I drove. For a few minutes, I considered driving off an embankment. This shocked me because I never had this feeling before and I knew it would be a selfish act, but I was exhausted and overwhelmed by my responsibility for Mom and was not thinking clearly. The interrupted sleep each night and a challenging job were also taking their toll on me. I was dashing home each day to make lunch for Mom and trying to keep many balls in the air the rest of the day at work.

I pulled into a parking lot and sat thinking about my situation. Then I thought about Mom. Who would take care of her? Then I thought about Dick, our children and our grandchildren. I was revived. Dick had always promised me that he would take care of Mom if anything happened to me because I couldn't count on my brother to help. I thought about my attitude. I decided I had an attitude problem. I needed to change it. I remembered Victor Frankl's book, *Man's Search for Meaning,* and how prisoners in concentration camps survived. The ones who lived through it had an attitude that they could be stripped of all human dignity but they couldn't be stripped of their attitude. It made them survivors. According to Frankl:

> We, who lived in concentration camps, can remember the men who walked through the huts comforting others, giving away their last piece of bread. They may have been few in number, but they offer sufficient proof that everything can be taken from a man but one thing: the last of the human freedoms to choose one's attitude in any given set of circumstances, to choose one's own way.

I said a prayer for help and guidance to help me survive this Alzheimer's onslaught, to help me be a survivor. Suddenly, I felt better. This was the beginning of a new attitude for me, actually a new-found peace too. I decided to be a survivor and not a victim. This was a good thing because Mom was entering the advanced stage of Alzheimer's disease.

The Advanced Stage

This stage is a series of losses. The loss of self is manifested by severe disorientation, lack of expression at times, delusions, little or no responsiveness and lack of purpose.

The most noticeable symptoms are physical. Alzheimer's victims may be unable to control bowel and bladder functions and unable to walk or talk. They may become apathetic, unable to communicate, and need 24 hour care.

Caregivers who provide 24 hour care during this stage often become socially isolated and are usually very sad to have lost the essence of their loved one's personhood. Some call it loss of self. The caregiver may suffer physical and emotional exhaustion as they witness their loved one deteriorating daily. The caregiver may also experience anticipatory grief.

If you are heading down the path of Alzheimer's, take heart. I'll share with you some of the positive things which happened as Mom and I took the path, especially since I changed my attitude.

The preceding stages are only approximate. Some say there are five stages. Whatever the number, it is a downhill course. Everyone is different and follows a different path. Denial of symptoms or cover up of symptoms may last longer in some families.

One thing is certain. Until there is a cure, there will be a downward path toward total dependency and death. Facing this, one must prepare.

12

Day Care

I took my Power in my Hand-
And went against the World-
'Twas not so much as David-had-
But I-was twice as bold-

I aimed my Pebble-but Myself
Was all the one that fell-
Was it Goliath-was too large-
Or was myself-too small?

—Emily Dickinson 1862

I arrive home from work and do not find the usual scene with Mom and Dick at the table, either talking or Mom is watching Dick reading the paper or doing a crossword puzzle. Today, Dick is sitting alone. He says softly, "Your mother is in her room with the door closed. You'd better check on her."

I run up the stairs with fleeting thoughts of what I will find. Is she ill? Not likely. She was fine at noon when I came home to fix her lunch. I relax a bit as I open the door. She is sound asleep. I walk softly to her bed and sit down next to her. She is so different in sleep than in her waking moments. She is breathing deeply with her mouth wide open. Her lips are sunken into her mouth as if the wind pressure of entering air has sucked the life out of her.

Her eyes open wide and I say, "Mom, I'm sorry. Did I wake you? Are you okay?"

"I fell down the stairs. I tripped, but I didn't want to bother you."

"Let's see."

I pull back the covers and see that her elbow is swollen many times over and is black and blue. I try to remain calm and say, "Mom, we need to get this checked out. Are you able to sit up?"

She flings her feet out of bed and sits up briskly to prove that she is okay, but she winces when she moves her arm. I can see that it is very painful.

I drive her to the emergency room. After a few hours and x-rays, we find that Mom's arm is broken and that she needs emergency surgery. A screw has to be placed in her elbow.

She does fine during the surgery and never complains of pain during her recuperation. This has been a pattern for the past few years. It seems as if her pain connections or pathways are severed by the disease. Now, I realize why she was able to go to sleep after breaking her arm. She feels no pain.

I, however, have the pain of guilt. If I hadn't been working, I would have been home and might have been able to prevent the accident or at least have been able to attend to her arm earlier. Slowly, I am beginning to acknowledge that Mom needs more supervision during the day.

As Mom's elbow heals, she spends more and more time in her chair looking out the window. No matter when I come home, she is there. When I suggest that she go to the Senior Center at least once a week, she says, "I don't want to go. I'm happy here."

I call several different agencies about alternatives. One day, as I am having my hair cut, the beautician tells me about her grandmother who had attended a day care center before going to a nursing home. She said that her grandmother was able to live at home longer because of the day care center. I ask the beautician for the name and location of the day care center. She gives them to me and even knows the phone number and a contact person. She adds, "The people are wonderful. My grandmother loved it."

I call the day care director the next day. She suggests that I visit the center with Mom and we schedule the time.

The center is clean and new and affiliated with a local hospital. The staff is caring and positive and treats everyone kindly and with respect. They all speak directly to Mom and not about her to me. The cost is similar to a child's day care, and like many working mothers, I need a loving place for my loved one. Mom needs more stimulation and this is a good alternative. Mom enjoyed her visit and the staff asks her to come back. She smiles and looks at me, "May I, Jennie?" I am relieved and make plans with the director.

Door to door transportation is provided for an additional cost. Even though it is expensive, the Center seems to be just what we need. Mom will have daily stimulation and company and I will get some relief. The bus will pick her up at 7:30 A.M. which is the time I leave for work. The bus will drop her off at 4:30 and Dick will be home by then. If he is detained, the bus driver will let Mom in the house. She needs a key on a string around her neck. She is a latch-key gramma. I worry about the security of our house when she has a key. I worry about the driver who will have access to our house key. I worry that Mom won't like the idea after a while.

Much to my surprise, Mom likes the idea of the bus. She thinks it's a good idea. She says, "You always do what's right for me." This is a major decision for Mom. I just hope it's the right decision.

To ease my mind, I take Mom to the day care the first day and stay several hours. It reminds me of the first day of kindergarten when I went with my children to ease my mind as well as to ease their transition.

Mom enjoys the company, the meals (breakfast and lunch), the activities, the music, and the rest period. Each person has their reclining chair and uses it after lunch while listening to restful music. Some people fall sound asleep. Not Mom. She closes her eyes and enjoys the music.

The worries about the bus driver are unfounded. He is trustworthy and very caring.

Everything is fine for several months. Then, winter approaches. The bus is an hour late one morning. I have to go to work and I can't leave her. If I leave her in the house with her coat, hat, and mittens, she probably won't answer the door when the driver comes and she will be alone and in her coat, hat, and mittens all day if he doesn't show up. She can't be alone all day any more. I wait with her after calling my office and explaining my dilemma. The bus had mechanical problems and another bus had to be located. That bus finally arrives two hours late.

It is impossible to get gloves on Mom's hands. She cannot comprehend matching the finger with the right slot in the glove. Mittens are much simpler and warmer. That's why young children wear them.

As winter settles in, the bus arrival is uncertain. The elderly people are no longer waiting outside for the bus. They also need more time to put on their heavy winter gear. This makes the route longer and the bus ride longer. Snow and ice also affect the ride time. My job is affected. I never know when I will be late. One thing is certain. Mom is not capable of being left alone. She no longer knows how to make a phone call and she needs 24/7 supervision.

Mom's increasing night wandering has caused her to be tired during the day. She is becoming very hard to arouse in the morning. Then, after eight months of day care, Mom says, "I don't think I need to go to work anymore." She thinks day care is her job. Now, she wants to quit her job. I need to respect her wishes.

I have some major decisions to make. The eight months of day care have been mostly wonderful for Mom and our family. Now, we have to make a change. Something has to give. I tell myself, "I'll think about it tomorrow."

13

Full-Time Care

The Service without Hope-
Is tenderest, I think-
Because 'tis unsustained
By stint-Rewarded Work-

Has impetus of Gain-
And impetus of Goal-
There is no Diligence like that
That knows not an Until-

—Emily Dickinson, 1863

I wait for the weekend when the pace slows down somewhat to talk with Dick. I share with him my frustrations and how the bus schedule is affecting my job. I tell him that no one at the office has complained but I have always prided myself on a job well done and I can't meet my own standards. I am exhausted. I get up from two to six times a night to help Mom back to bed. I weep as Dick holds me tight.

Dick says he realizes the stress I am feeling and asks me what I want to do. I say, "Retire and take care of Mom. I can't be up nights while she roams, and also, work days. I can't be late to work because of the bus schedule but I know I can't leave her alone. I know that I can't work and take care of Mom. She's beginning to complain. We both are too tired for the present situation."

Dick says, "Okay, retire. I know you love your job so this must be important to you." He takes my hand and squeezes it. We sit quietly for a few minutes. Then, I say, "Can we afford it?" Dick says, "We'll manage." I know that this decision will make a big difference in our income. I also know my priority. Dad taught me well. I feel no resentment about the decision. On the contrary, I feel some peace in making the right decision for me. I think about other caregivers who don't have a supportive spouse or family or who can't afford day care or to be a full-time caregiver. I have a lot to be thankful for.

I go to the Superintendent of the school district where I work and tell him the whole story, tears and all. He is very understanding and suggests several alternatives: job sharing, a year's leave of absence, part-time, etc. I feel reaffirmed by his caring and understanding and faith in my competence. I am especially touched by his humanity. This is the type of person who serves children well. His priorities are in order.

Dick and I review the alternatives until late in the night. We both agree that a full retirement is the best option especially since Mom is still night-stalking. We don't know how long she will need care. We would have to hire someone to help if I continued to work and we feel we would be the best help. I am very tired and need to make a change so we decide on retirement. We do not consider a nursing home because we do not want that option. We never want that option. We realize that a nursing home may be the best option down the road, but we want to care for her as long as we are able.

14

Time Away

Rests at Night
The Sun from shining,
Nature-and some Men-
Rest at Noon-some Men-
While Nature
And the Sun-go on-

—Emily Dickinson, 1863

The whole family decides to go to the lake house in Wisconsin. This house is like a retreat for Dick, Mom, and me. It is in a small town on a lake about two hours away. This is to be my first trip since my retirement.

The feeling is that of a child on a bike with the whole day to squander. The wind is blowing my hair and I can pedal fast or slow depending on my moods. The thrill of the moment is intoxicating.

I set out in the car with Mom beside me. Dick couldn't come at the last minute because he had to work on Saturday for the first time in many, many years. I have finally retired and Dick is more involved than ever in his job.

I don't dwell on Dick's absence. I miss him. He can laugh with me or give me a knowing look when Mom does something bizarre. This includes the time Mom smeared her feces all over the bathroom curtains when she ran out of toilet paper or when she shredded her diaper all over the dining room. These moments are the epoxy bonding us forever as partners in life experiences known only by sharing of life's basic functions.

I am appreciative of the mature love which has developed between Dick and me. I remember the early years of intense passion, possessiveness, love, jealousy, and excitement. Now, there is peace, deep trust, an even deeper love, and the excitement is just being together. The passion remains. My one hope is that my children also will experience such a mature love, but without the heartaches Dick and I share watching Mom's decline.

It was as if I were setting off on a journey by myself. My companion, Mom, doesn't know her name, her address, or what day it is. She knows only that I am happy and she reflects my feeling. It reminds me of young mothers who talk about their babies being upset when the mothers are tired and cranky and the babies appear happy when the mothers are happy. Babies pick up the cues from their mothers. Now Mom is picking up my cues. She laughs as we drive out of the driveway. It is a laughter of empty thoughts. It is, however, better than anger or tears.

We reach the Wisconsin border and the highway has a 65 MPH limit. I turn on the cruise control, put on a tape of hymns for Mom, and take a mental holiday with thoughts of a weekend of rest and renewal. After all, I don't have to go to work on Monday and I always feel a sense of excitement when I am going to see my children and grandchildren.

The grandchildren rush out to greet us with hugs and kisses. They are the treasures of a long life. Their parents are next in line. The porch is filled with balloons which say, "Happy Retirement" and a five foot long banner with "Happy Retirement, Mom" on it. My eyes fill with tears of happiness

I realize that retirement, for me, means retirement from a good paying job and a transfer into a full-time job of loving, supporting, trying to understand and endure life with Mom and her Alzheimer's disease. There will no longer be a regular pay check for services rendered, no evaluation of performance, no sense of progress, only gradual decline.

Retirement does mean more time with my family and, maybe, some more personal time. I realize that I haven't had personal time since Mom needed supervision. I have been getting my hair cut only when it is obviously too long and uneven. I shave only my lower legs in the winter when a swim suit isn't a consideration. I shop for clothes only when a special occasion arises and these excursions usually take place an hour before closing time. While I am relieved to have found something to wear, I never feel a real satisfaction with what I have found. I never have time for a fragrant and leisurely bath. I do take quick daily showers. I wonder if this is what a working caregiver's life is like for others as well.

The day is filled with the squeals of young children experiencing delight with new-found water skills. Ryan, our grandson, swims under water with his eyes closed, and is driven to practice his new skills. Jamie, our granddaughter, discovers she can stay afloat if she kicks her feet. I feel a release in seeing their progress and being a part of it. Then, I look up at the porch and see Mom sitting hour after hour almost in a stupor, separated from the vibrant life around her.

Jeff is making a fishing lure with future plans to catch a big one. Blake garners competence in the water as he watches his older cousin, Ryan. Blake tries to imitate Ryan's success. He is intent on achievement. Krissy, our granddaughter, rides astride a large inflated alligator, a Cleopatra of the sandbox, just content with her power to see and be a two-year-old with a new world opening up for her every minute.

It is all so exciting that I run up to the porch to get Mom to come down and see it all. We put a bench at the top of the stairs leading to the beach where she has a good view of all the activities on this beautiful summer day. Everyone goes back to their summer fun. It's our way of including Mom, even as a spectator.

A few minutes go by and I look up toward the bench. Mom is gone. Laurie, my daughter, calls to me. Mom is found in a fetal position near the porch. Laurie asks her if everything is okay. She says, "Yes." Laurie lovingly helps her grandmother get up and walks slowly with her, reassuring her with every step. Laurie hugs her grandmother when they reach the porch.

These are moments which I savor. Someone else is sharing Mom's care, even if only for a brief moment. Warm feelings for my daughter flood my thoughts. I vow at that moment not to be her burden in my old age.

This is the ambivalence of care. I've seen it many times before with parents of disabled children. They toil endlessly caring for their special children, but do not want their other children to ever experience what they have gone through. It's not because their other children don't have the capacity. They generally have more to give because of their experience with their sibling's disabilities, but some resentment is probably inevitable, no matter how much the special child is loved. I am slowly beginning to deal with my own resentment by acknowledging it. This resentment is because of the situation. I am pained by the situation Mom is in. I am angry at God. Is this God's plan for her? My pain is so great for her that I would trade places with her to free her of Alzheimer's disease. I ask not, "Why me?" but "Why her?"

The day ends with a picnic on the porch with everyone looking cleansed by a day in the water, everyone but Mom. Her face is filled with wrinkles and she is white as a white sheet. She eats sparingly and seems miles away in her thoughts. Every time someone laughs, she laughs and then retreats into her "Winds of Yesterday."

The sunset over the lake has a calming influence on everyone, young and old alike. Mom yawns and says she is going to bed. I follow her to the bedroom and help her dress for bed. She starts to put the arms of her nightgown on her legs. I lost it! I say, "Mom, don't you know that this sleeve is for your arm?" She kisses my hands and says, "I love you. You'll get your reward someday." Mom's unconditional love is her greatest gift. I was wrong for being so impatient. I weep inwardly and say a short prayer for patience and forgiveness.

I put on her adult diapers and she says, "You treat me like a baby." I say, "Mom, I don't know what else to do." She says, "Thanks." This surprises me. Maybe she has pleasant memories of the love and care given to babies. To her, it may have been a sign of deep love. I hope. This incident helps me realize that Mom should not be treated like a baby. A baby couldn't interpret the incident the way Mom did. She is an adult with many life experiences and I should talk to her with this in mind. It will help maintain her dignity. I will no longer treat her like a baby. I will treat her like an adult who has special needs.

I tuck her into bed and go downstairs to savor some hours with no responsibility. It is not long before my eyes become heavy. My personal time is becoming less and less. I have to sleep when she sleeps and it is an interrupted sleep at that.

I climb the stairs and crawl into the other bed in mom's room. I usually sleep with Dick, but since he isn't here and more beds are needed than we have, I decide to sleep in the room with Mom. I turn on the night light in the room. Mom looks so little and frail but peaceful as she sleeps.

About 1 A.M., I am awakened by a shuffling noise. Mom is roaming around the room gently caressing each item on the bookcase and in the room. She is making a throaty sound when she exhales. There is no sound when she inhales. Her gown is covered with urine and feces on the back. I can see in the dim light that her bed is wet and discolored.

I get out of bed and ask her if she needs anything. She looks at me with vacant and wide eyes. There is no sense of recognition. It is almost as if she is hypnotized. I am unable to bring her out of this state. I walk with her to the bathroom.

When we reach the toilet, she sits down. She doesn't pull her diapers down. I reach to pull them down. She grabs my arm and says, "God damn" in a loud voice, and tries to bite my arm. I am scared of my own mother. I have never seen Mom like this. She has always told us, "People who use swear words lack the vocabulary to express themselves in any other way." Not only is the swearing unlike Mom, but the physical aggression is unlike her. She didn't believe in spanking us as children. She believed in "time out." She said physical aggression was not a way to teach others, only a way to get rid of one's own frustrations. Years later, we gave her a large punching clown and she laughed and said that was a better way to get rid of frustrations because no one else was hurt.

I wonder if she had many nights like this where she stalked the room and went "wild" by moonlight. I have been up with her at night many times before, but I never witnessed what went on in her bedroom behind closed doors. Her private hell in her mind is probably being relived every night.

The next morning, Mom awakes refreshed. I am exhausted because she was up four times. It's like a new mother who gets up for night feedings with a baby. The baby wakes up cheerful and gurgling. The mother is worn out by the interrupted sleep but is revived by the baby's smile. Only in this case, I am worn out and the mother doesn't remember the night. I am somewhat revived by her smile. I remember that she's not a baby.

15

An Alternative to Care

What I can do-I will-
Though it be little as a Daffodil-
That I cannot-must be
Unknown to possibility-

—Emily Dickinson, 1862

The summer is pleasant even though Dick has to work seven days a week. The grandchildren come over or we go to the lake for a diversion.

By late autumn, Mom has lost not only her short-term memory but her long-term memory as well. She tells grandiose stories of trips to Europe even though she has never been there. She doesn't remember Dad, her husband of 53 years. Her eyes have a vacant look when I mention his name. She has no recognition of Dick, her son, or her grandchildren, or her great-grandchildren. She still recognizes me. I am her connection to the world. I feel privileged, but overwhelmed and sad at the same time.

I am up several times during the night in order to settle her back in bed after a wandering episode. I am so tired all day but I can't take a nap because, like a 2 year-old, she can't be left without supervision. She would eat raw rice, coffee grounds, or anything else in the kitchen. I take the knobs off of the cook top so she won't start a fire. She can't be trusted with the grandchildren around. So, leaving her with our children and grandchildren is not something I have asked of them. One time, Mom grabbed our two-year-old granddaughter's dress and wouldn't let go. Mom kept twisting the dress and pulling it. Her eyes looked vicious. Poor Mollie screamed with fright. I don't blame her. I've had that feeling. I quickly rescued Mollie's dress from Mom.

One day, a friend called and said that they have a lady working for them who is available for the weekend. They say that the lady is caring, reliable, and trustworthy. Dick and I think this would be a good opportunity to go to the lake house or take a romantic getaway, our first since Mom's diagnosis. We would only be two hours away if something comes up. I am mainly looking forward to sleeping through the night. My needs are simple: rest and sleep.

For a trial run, we go out to dinner on Friday night and come home early just to see how things are going. We arrive to a cold house. Mom has turned the thermostat so the heat went off. The lady didn't know anything about thermostats. They did, however, get along fine otherwise.

We happily prepare to leave the next morning. We cover the thermostat with masking tape. We lock our bedroom because Mom would take things and hide them. We give the lady our phone number and leave.

Dick and I sleep late on Sunday morning. Dick makes his delicious Swedish pancakes. It is about noon when we finish doing the dishes. We read for awhile, take a long walk, talk with no interruptions, and go grocery shopping. It has been a long time since we went shopping together because one of us had to "baby-sit" Mom. It's a reminder to be grateful for the little things in life. I will never take shopping with Dick for granted again.

I tell Dick that I will make him a special dinner. We shower and have a glass of wine and then, I fix dinner. Dick lounges on the couch and watches T.V. We are peacefully happy.

After breakfast on Sunday, we head for home. We discover that Mom has locked the guest bedroom where the lady was going to sleep so she didn't have a bed. Not only that, she didn't have a blanket or a pillow. She spent the cold winter's night on a sofa covered only by her coat. She informs me that Mom has not eaten since we left because Mom doesn't like her cooking.

Dick and I finally admit that Mom's care is engulfing us. She has been with us for many years and it has been our privilege to have her in our home, but now we need help to provide her with 24 hour care. We are going to investigate our alternatives.

A few months later, we drive up North for a winter weekend with Mom. Dick makes a fire in the fireplace and we sit and watch the dancing flames and read the papers. I see an advertisement about a new Community Based Residential Facility (CBRF) for the elderly in the town near our lake home. It is a group home for elderly folks who cannot take care of themselves and who need 24-hour care and supervision, but do not need a nursing home.

The next morning, Mom, Dick, and I visit the CBRF. It is an answer to our prayers. Mom would have 24 hour care. We could bring her home for visits. She would have the company of her peers and a full day of activities as well. Dick and

I would get some much needed relief and I would get some much needed sleep. Mom likes the idea. She thinks she is buying her own room. She thinks she is gaining independence. She is constantly worried that she is a burden. We reassure her that she is not and that we love her and we will see her often.

We check with neighbors about the CBRF. We check the background of the caregiver, a longtime nurse. We check with the city on licensing. These are things you would check on if your child was going to a daycare center or a nursery school. You have to be your child's advocate just as I am Mom's advocate. Everything checks out well.

I take Mom to the doctor for a physical exam which is required by the CBRF and she qualifies for entry. After a few weeks, all arrangements are made and she moves into a private room. The cost is about half the cost of a nursing home. The CBRF seems to offer her some independence. I believe that many people are in nursing homes when they could be in less restrictive environments such as the CBRF. My state of Illinois does not have CBRFs, unfortunately. The CBRF provides a bridge between the home and the nursing home. The home atmosphere is very comforting to Mom.

Two weeks after Mom entered the CBRF, the nurse/owner calls me to say that Mom has a prolapsed uterus. I take her to the doctor who says that Mom needs a hysterectomy. The doctor attempts to explain the surgery to Mom. After his fifth attempt, I tell him that I will take care of it. Mom has a complete vaginal hysterectomy. She is a wild woman for a week after surgery due to the effects of the anesthesia. The hospital staff ties Mom's hands. She begs me to untie them which I do. This was a big mistake. She starts throwing things and tries to get out of bed. The nurses quickly tie her up again. She calms down after a week and goes back to the CBRF.

Mom makes a good adjustment and we see her frequently. I drive up three times during the week and Dick and I go up on weekends. It is a four hour drive but we want to keep in close touch. It's too bad that Illinois doesn't have this kind of care. Illinois has "assisted living" but most of them house many people and lack the close supervision of the type Mom requires.

Six months go by and we receive a letter from the owner about Mom:

> Dear Jennie,
>
> I'm sorry that my phone conversations are so short and uninformative, but with the listening ears and interruptions that are around here, it's difficult to be detailed.
>
> As far as Cleo's condition: one of the biggest problems we have is because of her being so hard of hearing. More times than not, when someone speaks,

she misunderstands it. With this, a domino effect happens with persons having the conversation. When the person spoken to, answers, she accuses them of interrupting. We feel that a hearing aid would be very worthwhile.

The severe confusion she was having has lessened, but we continue to see her Dementia increasing. Her intellectual faculties are inane when it comes to activities of daily living; dressing, making the bed, using condiments, moving bedroom furniture, use of toilet paper, use of clothing, use of towels etc..

She does continue to go in other resident's rooms and remove their personal belongings.

Her personality varies. Usually she's very pleasant and polite. She continues with small outbursts at times. These are usually caused by her misunderstanding. Some personality changes we realize are due to her Dementia. Her phobia of people looking in her bedroom window continues.

We will continue to monitor her condition and to care for her as long as we can. We've grown to love her as one of the family. I'll update you if there are any changes.

Sincerely

Mom is examined and fitted with two hearing aids. There is a slight improvement in her hearing apparently. We're not sure how a valid test could be done on Mom. Keeping track of the hearing aids is a major problem. She takes them off and hides them. She takes the batteries out of them at times. Nothing is ever simple with Mom.

After a year at the CBRF, I receive a letter from the owner saying that Mom requires too much care and should be placed in a nursing home. I thought Mom's care was finally stable for a while, but, once again, it's not. Such is the emotional roller coaster that goes with Alzheimer's disease.

16

The Search for a Nursing Home

What Inn is this
Where for the night
Peculiar Traveler comes?
Who is the Landlord?
Where the maids?
Behold, what curious rooms!
No ruddy fires on the hearth-
No brimming Tankards flow-
Necromancer! Landlord!
Who are these below?

—Emily Dickinson, 1859

Dick and I begin the arduous and emotional task of finding a nursing home. Our hearts are very heavy because we had hoped that Mom would live out her days in the CBRF. But that is not to be.

I call several agencies, talk to friends, doctors, and others. We compile a list of recommended nursing homes within a 30 mile radius of our home. We visit all of them.

The home which is closest to our village was written up in the local paper as a place where neglect of patients has allegedly occurred. It is a beautiful new facility but the neglect charges scare us.

We visit one home which is the cheapest on our list. When we enter the front door, we are overcome by the smell of urine and feces. The floors are dirty and the residents are lined up in wheel chairs in the hall. I start gagging from the stench and the horror of people living like this. We quickly leave.

Many of the nursing homes have Alzheimer's units. We feel Mom would rather be integrated with other patients. Finally, after an exhaustive search, we find a nursing home which offers excellent care, activities, is clean and has a competent and sociable staff. They talk to the residents rather than about them. They call them by name. All of the residents appear well-cared for. Their hair is clean and combed. They welcome family visitors and the Alzheimer's patients are integrated, not set apart in a separate unit. The cost is higher than most nursing homes. Medicare does not pay for custodial care for AD patients in a nursing home. We know this is going to be costly but Mom deserves the best care we can find and afford.

We take Mom to visit the nursing home twice and she seems content there. Just as if she is going to camp, we get her special clothes. Sweat suits are recommended as well as shoes with Velcro fasteners or slip-ons. We put name labels on her things and pack her bags.

Mom has been at home for two weeks since she left the CBRF. During that time, she has almost fallen down the stairs, has wandered outside and got lost in the woods, has tried to eat kitchen cleanser, and is still wandering half the night. I am terrified to leave her alone. My bathroom trips are very short.

Mom no longer uses flatware. She eats with her fingers. She resists taking a shower or bath and has to be bribed with candy. She still takes our things and hides them. We nearly go crazy trying to find her hiding places for her hearing aids. She flushed one down the toilet and we had to get a replacement.

It is with mixed feelings that we take Mom to the nursing home. We are both exhausted and frustrated but also, deeply saddened. I am also disappointed in myself that I am unable to care for Mom for the rest of her life in our home. I finally accept the fact that I can't do it. The only consolation is that the CBRF could no longer care for her, even with day and night staff. We were able to care for Dick's Mom with cancer until her death but Alzheimer's disease is different. It has been eight years and we are sadly crying "Uncle," the cry of surrender.

We drive slowly to the nursing home when the day comes for her to go. I hate the thought of another change for Mom.

The staff at the nursing home is wonderful. They get Mom involved in a sing-a-long activity and suggest that we say our good-byes. Mom continues singing as we kiss and hug her and leave. We glance back through our tears to see her singing, "Let Me Call You Sweetheart" with gusto. Music has always given Mom pleasure and, surprisingly, she remembers most of the old songs of her yester-years.

Since Mom no longer recognizes me or anyone else, anyone can substitute. This is bittersweet. It makes it easier for us to leave, but it is sad to think that she doesn't know she is moving. I would be very unsettled to find myself in such a foreign world, but to Mom, it is home if the people are kind and caring, whoever they are.

Dick and I have tears all the way home. Sometimes life just isn't fair. We know that, but it pains us when life does not seem fair to a sweet little lady who loves everyone.

Mom spends a year and a half in the nursing home. She seems content and well-cared for. I visit her daily. She says, "Here's the nice lady." When I do something for her like combing her hair or giving her a massage, she says, "You'll get your reward." It won't be her money because it's all gone. I know it'll be something very special.

A caregiver's life isn't finished when the loved one enters a nursing home. I pick up her dirty laundry and take it home to wash it. I attend staff conferences on Mom's care and progress. I feed her lunch which takes about an hour. She eats only pureed foods. Sometimes, I gag when I smell cabbage pureed. I take Mom to McDonald's everyday for ice cream. She loves ice cream. When I leave to go, I hug and kiss her and she says, "Goodbye nice lady." I miss being "Sister."

There are a series of staff changes at the nursing home. I notice that Mom has become agitated. She starts striking out at other residents, scratching or hitting them. The new head nurse brings her dog to work everyday. Mom is allergic to it and she starts wheezing. Instead of keeping the dog away from her, Mom is given inhalers several times a day. The nursing home staff's response to Mom's agitation is to medicate her more. The monthly medication bill is staggering. She is becoming very groggy. She also seems to need more attention than she is getting. We are reminded that a caregiver's most important role in the nursing home scene is that of an advocate. Mom is spending most of the time in bed wheezing. She's agitated because she can't breathe. The new staff aren't like the old staff and the remaining old staff have low morale. We have to do something.

About this time, a new CBRF opens in Wisconsin and Dick and I go to the grand opening. It's a few minutes from our lake home. There are 16 resident rooms, all private and beautifully decorated. There is a large staff, activities, home cooked meals, and a family atmosphere. Mostly though, we are impressed with the Director, Ruby. She is a short, tiny-boned bundle of energy and kindness. She knows how to listen. We share our concerns with Ruby. We are worried that Mom will not be accepted because of her behaviors. Ruby suggests that we bring Mom for a visit.

We take Mom for a visit and she wants to stay. She can't though until she has a physical exam and an interview with the county health nurse. We schedule these appointments and we pray that she'll be accepted. We are not optimistic because we don't know of many people who go from a nursing home to a CBRF. Usually, it's the other way around. We get a phone call from Ruby. Mom is accepted. Yes, life is fair at times.

We buy her a new bedroom set, a lamp that lights when you touch it, and a picture. Mom never understands the lamp mechanism. So it has to be unplugged.

Mom thoroughly enjoys her stay at "Ruby's Place" as she calls it. The homey atmosphere is comfortable for Dick and me. We become part of the family there.

Mom's first year there is uneventful in a good sort of way. Soon Mom will celebrate her 90th birthday. All is right in the world. Life is good except for the AD. We are blessed to have Ruby and her staff.

We are well aware that Ruby sets the tone for care. Ruby is always well-dressed and groomed and she has a special attitude toward the elderly. The poem which follows reminds me of Ruby:

BEATITUDES FOR THE AGING

Blessed are they who understand
My faltering steps and palsied hand.
Blessed are they who know my ears today
Must strain to catch the words they say.
Blessed are they who seem to know that my eyes
Are dim and my wits are slow.
Blessed are they who look away when coffee
Spilled on the table today.
Blessed are they with a cheery smile that stops to
Chat for a little while.
Blessed are they who never say, "You've told that story
Twice today."
Blessed are they who know the ways to bring back
Memories of yesterdays.
Blessed are they who make it known
That I'm loved, respected and not alone.
Blessed are they who know I'm at a loss

To find the strength to carry my cross.
Blessed are they who ease the days
On my journey Home in loving ways.

—Author Unknown

I think there should be Academy Awards, not for acting, but for being REAL, for being humane, for being special. Ruby would get one.

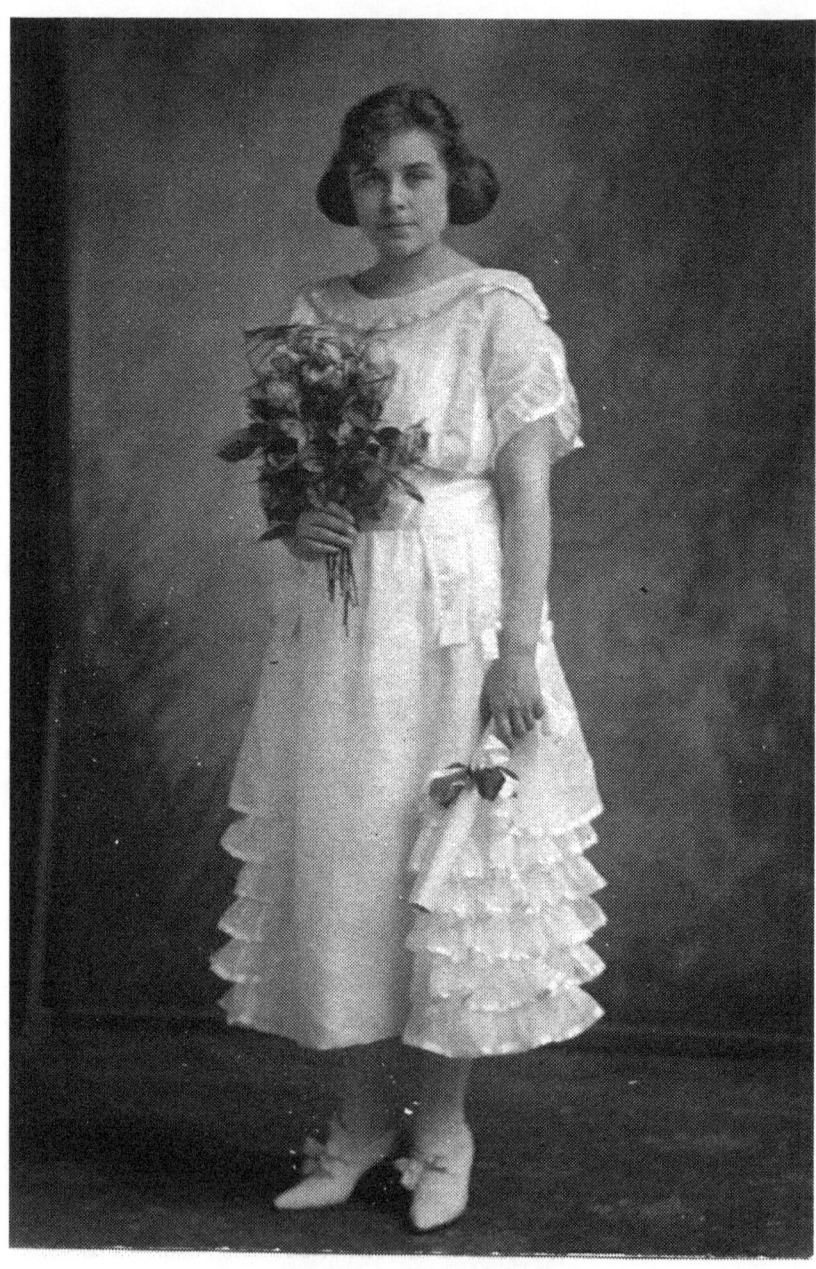

1. Cleo As A High School Graduate

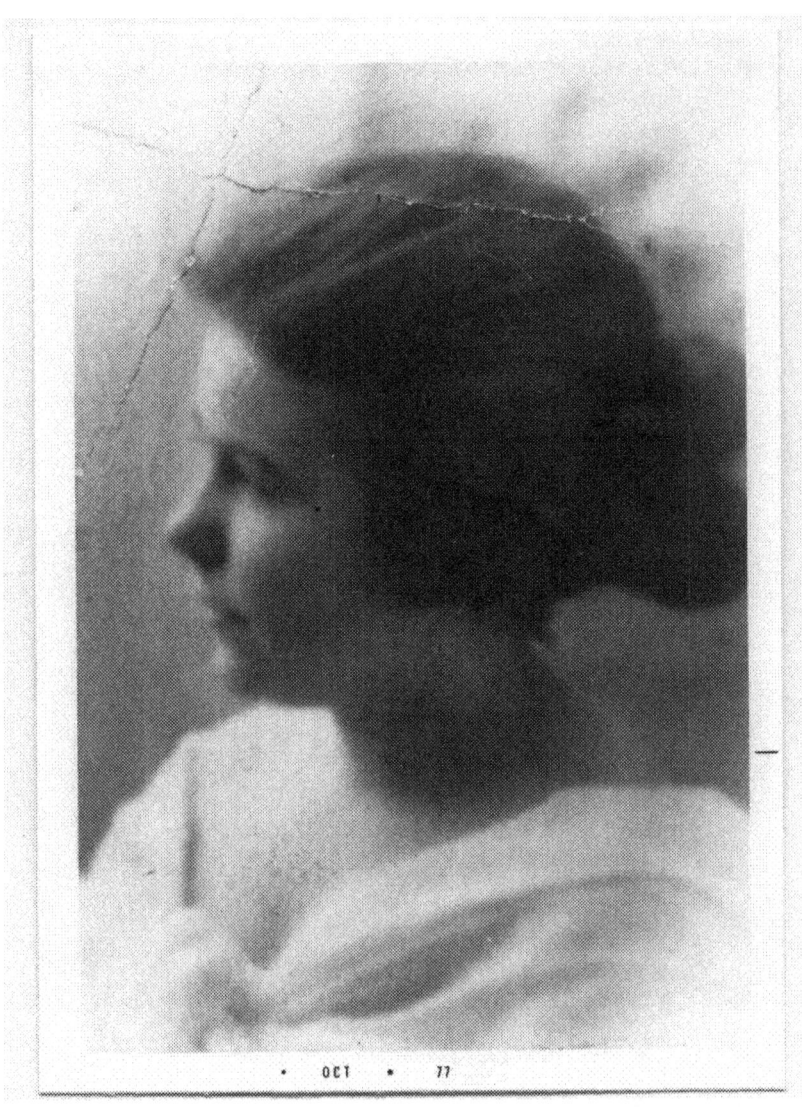

2. Cleo As A Young Woman

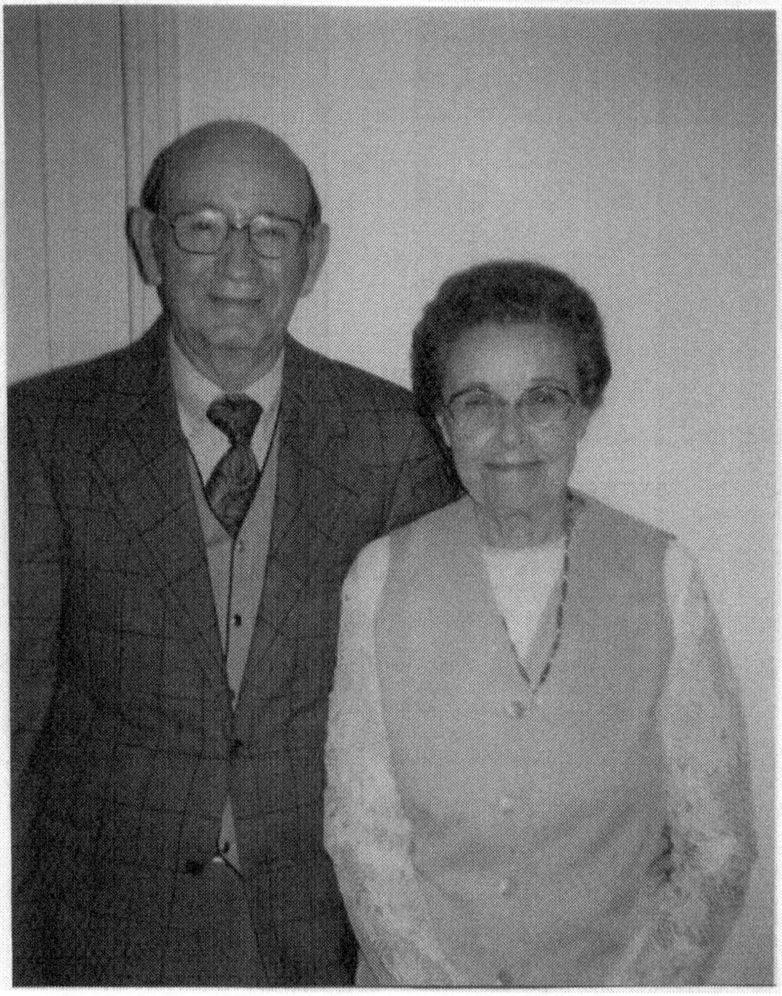

3. Cleo and Her Husband of 53 Years

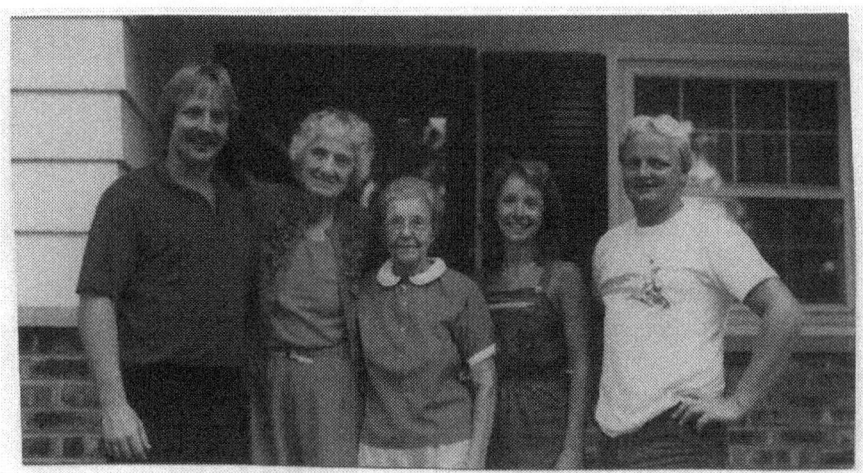

4. Cleo with Helen and Their Grandchildren

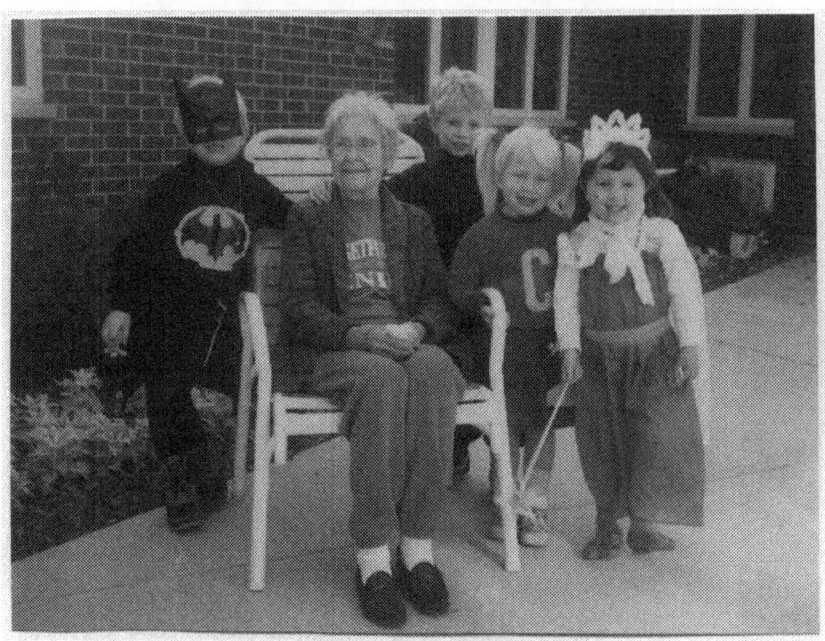

5. Cleo and Her Great-grandchildren

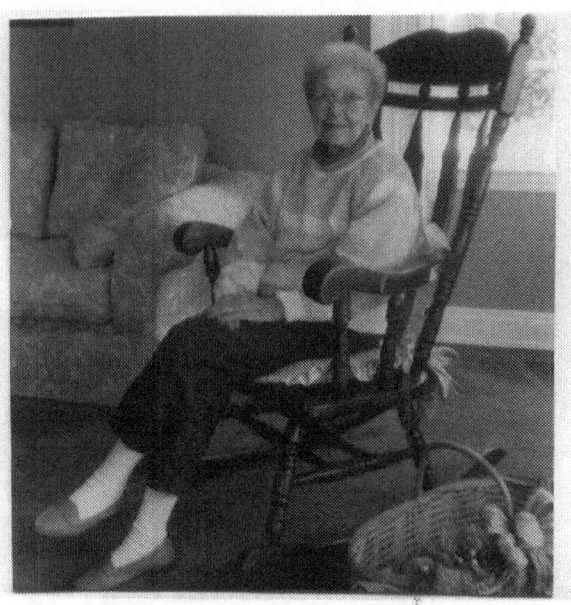

6. Cleo in Her Rocking Chair

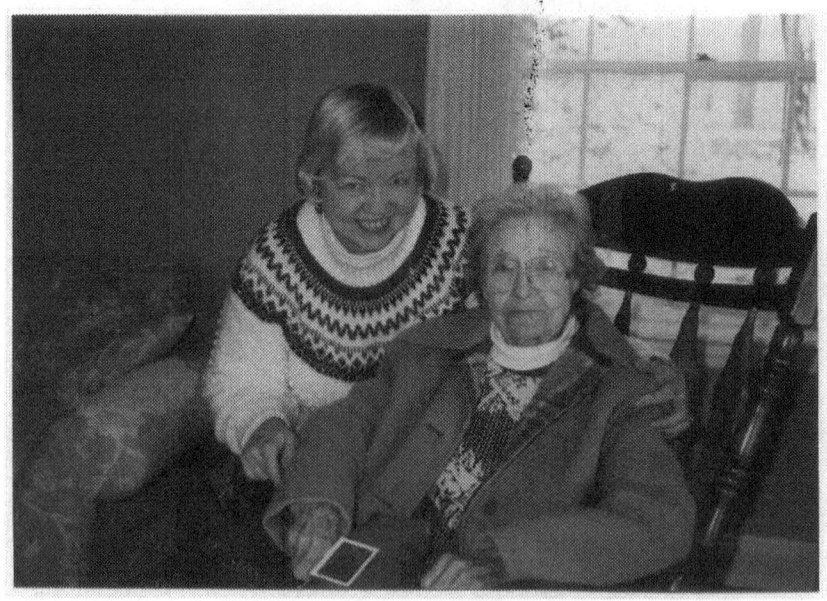

7. Cleo and Sister

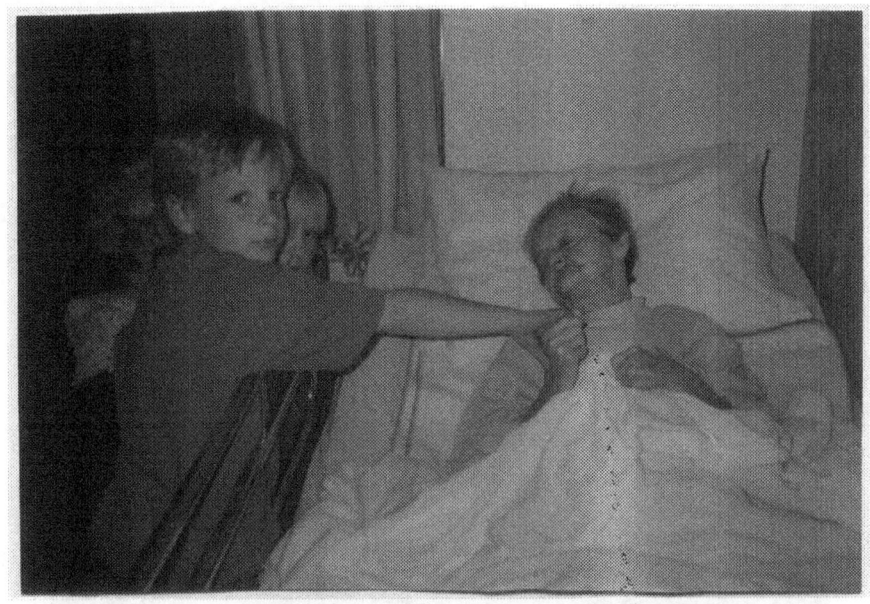

8. Cleo Saying Goodbye to the Great-grand-children

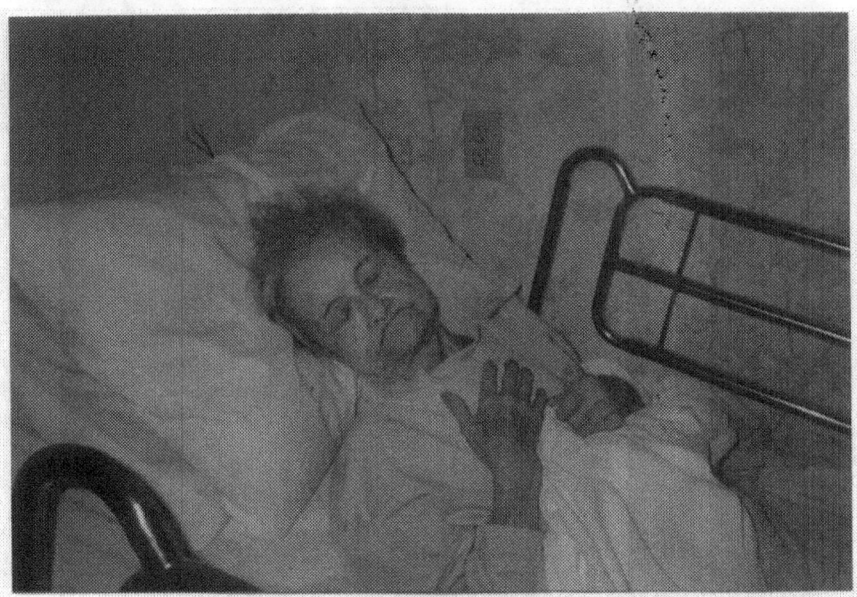

9. Cleo's Last Days

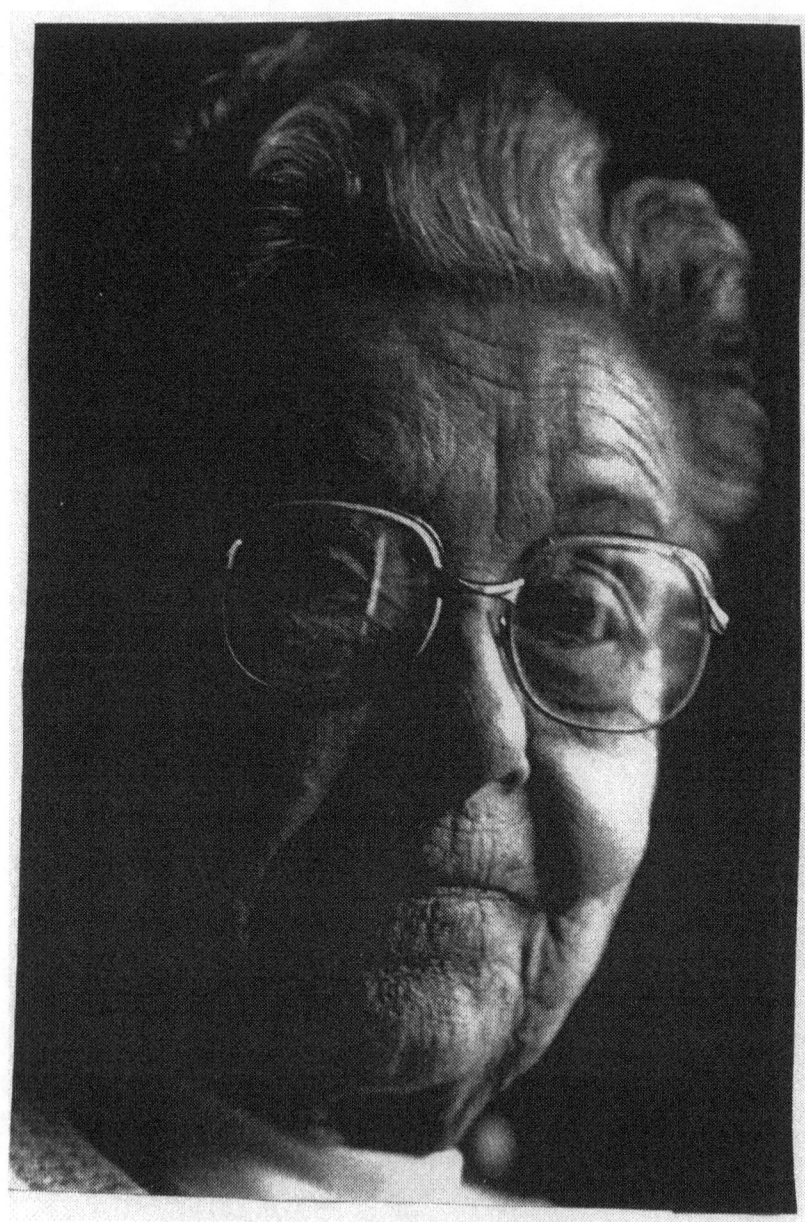

10. Memories Are A Precious Gift

17

90TH Birthday Party

I shall know why-when Time is over-
And I have ceased to wonder why-
Christ will explain each separate anguish
In the fair schoolroom of the sky-

He will tell me what "Peter" promised-
And I-for wonder at his woe-
I shall forget the drop of Anguish
That scalds me now-that scalds me now!

—Emily Dickinson, 1860

Mom is going to be 90 years old on Monday, August 31st. I call Ruby.

"You know, it's Mom's birthday on Monday."

"Yes, I have it on the calendar."

"Would it be all right if I bring cake and punch for a party Monday afternoon?"

"Sure, that would be fine. By the way, I need a check for $25 for a permanent."

"I'll bring it tomorrow."

"Thanks."

"See you then."

I hang up the phone and then think about the whole situation. Mom doesn't know she'll be 90. She doesn't even know the date of her birthday. She still won't know when we have the party. She doesn't have a past anymore that she remembers. She doesn't think about the future. She only has now, the immediate, just like an infant. It's a true existential existence. The point is, when the party occurs, it'll be now and now is all she has. Why not party!

I think maybe it's guilt that makes me plan a party. My mother is 90 years old. There should be some rite of passage, some acknowledgement of her life, her longevity and her accomplishments. If she doesn't have the brain power to understand the importance of her life, who will? We will. Mom loves a party, especially the singing and the cake. We will celebrate.

My brother may or may not send her a card. He stopped sending her presents long ago. His daughter (Mom's granddaughter) calls long distance to find out her birth date. Maybe she'll send a card.

Dick and I go to the store and buy balloons and I bake a sheet cake and write, "Happy Birthday, Cleo" on top. I place two candles, a nine and a zero, on top. We are all set except for the drink. We stop and get four cans of fruit punch. Dick puts the cake on the back floor of the car and the rest of the party goods in the trunk and we're on our way.

We walk into the CBRF with all the goodies. I see Mom. She looks regal with her new permanent and her pink outfit. Her head is slightly lowered as if she is about to nod off.

As we approach, she looks at us with vacant eyes. I say, "Happy Birthday, Mom" and I wrap my arms around her for a warm hug. She looks at me and then at Dick and lowers her head again and closes her eyes.

We pour the red fruit punch into the glasses, cut the cake into squares, put a party hat on each person, and give each a balloon. I hear one lady scream and I turn around to see that she has spilled the red fruit punch all over the carpeted floor. She keeps repeating, "Look what I did." I say, "Don't worry. I'll clean it up." I'm thinking I should have brought lemonade or a punch which wasn't red.

I go to the kitchen for some rags and start wiping up the punch. It is so hot in the room that my face is turning red as I blot the carpet. Dick helps and Ruby puts "Beer Barrel Polka" into the tape player. They all sit with their hats, balloons and punch and watch expressionless. As I get up off the floor, I see Mom digging into the cake with her fingers leaving tracks across the frosting. Her mouth is covered with frosting.

We start singing, "Happy Birthday" and almost everyone joins in. I say most everyone because one lady says she is dizzy and goes to bed. A gentleman says he doesn't want to come to the party and continues to watch TV in another room. One lady throws her balloon at Dick in an apparent effort to relate to him. He bats the balloon back and she squeals with delight each time she bats the balloon. This reminds me of birthday parties for toddlers. They love balloons but you have to be careful because they can be dangerous to toddlers.

Then a lovely lady in purple says, "We haven't sung, 'Happy Birthday'." So, we sing it again. Every few minutes, she says, "We haven't sung 'Happy Birthday'." We sing it again. I lost count after singing it six times.

A ninety-seven year-old lady in a wheelchair decides to bat her balloon. Only, she has a glass of red punch in her hand. And yes, she spills the red liquid all over herself, the wheelchair, and the rug. Dick gets down on the floor and begins blotting and then scrubbing the rug. I wipe off the ladies clothes and now, it feels like a hundred degrees in here. Homes for the elderly are usually kept quite warm because the elderly are often cold.

We finish opening the presents. I say "we" because Mom couldn't figure out how to unwrap the gifts. So, Dick and I open them. There is no recognition that the gift is hers or that she is the only one with presents. She just lowers her head and promptly falls asleep.

Dick and I clean up the plates and glasses and announce, "Thanks for coming." We have the feeling that, if we don't bring closure, the rest of the residents would continue to sit and stare vacantly. Slowly, the group disperses with Ruby's help. One of the ladies takes a piece of cake to the gentleman watching TV. He comes over to Mom, takes her hand, shakes it, and says, "Happy Birthday. Thank you very much."

One lady murmurs softly, "He's the most polite person here."

As we get in the car to go home, Dick and I heave a sigh and talk about what might have been. We both have a feeling of "What's the use?" Mom no longer has fun at a party. She doesn't understand what is happening. The presents were forgotten immediately. Mom seems to thrive on consistency and the party is almost like an intrusion into the security of her world where sameness is comfortable. We have learned a lesson though. Sameness is good for AD victims. It's a form of reassurance when everything else is in chaos. Dick turns to me and says, "You're a good daughter." It was enough. My mood lightened.

18

A Broken Bone

For each ecstatic instant
We must an anguish pay
In keen and quivering ratio
To the ecstasy.

For each beloved hour
Sharp pittances of years-
Bitter contested farthings-
And Coffers heaped with Tears!

—(Excerpt from "For each ecstatic instant")
Emily Dickinson, 1859

Mom is doing well in Ruby's Place. She loves Ruby, the staff, and the other residents. One initial problem seems to be solved. The residents sit up until 8:30 or 9 o'clock in the evening and awake about 7 A.M. After lunch, a lot of the residents take a nap. Mom never took a nap in the past for as long as I can remember and she doesn't take one now. Over a period of weeks, Mom became sleep deprived.

She begins to wander into other resident's rooms "borrowing" their things and is irritable, even hostile at times. Ruby decides to see what would happen if Mom is allowed to sleep until she wakes up in the morning. The first morning, Mom sleeps until 2:30 in the afternoon. The staff looks in on her often. For several days, Mom sleeps late in the morning. As she becomes more rested, her mood improves and her wandering decreases. She still doesn't take naps during the day. She just sleeps later. She stills wakes up several times during the night and wanders. The night staff watches over her wanderings.

Things are better for Mom now. She seems happy. The staff is caring and upbeat. I still have the responsibility for Mom, but it is shared with people I trust. For the first time, I feel I can relax and reach out to others outside the family and maybe have some fun.

I talk with my old high school friends. We graduated in 1949 and 1950. There are seven of us who have kept in touch. We make plans to have an old-fashioned slumber party, just like the ones we used to have. I invite them to the lake home for the weekend.

I breathe in the heady smells of summer, marvel at my roses, and feel healed by the warmth of the summer sun. I think, "Life is good."

The slumber party gives me a new focus. I read gourmet cookbooks and magazines in preparation for the meals with old friends. I think of fun, sun, and "catching up." I locate some audio tapes of music in the 50's. As I listen to them, I remember easier times when my overriding concerns were what to wear to the Casbah (the high school dance club), what college to attend, and whether I should cut my hair or let it grow.

Then, Ruby calls and says, "Your Mom fell out of bed and broke her arm. She's okay. She's in the hospital and will be there a day or two. By the way, we drove her to the hospital. We thought an ambulance might further upset her and would cost more. I'll go see her tonight." Ruby's an angel.

I say, "Ruby, Thanks. I'll drive up. I'll be there in two hours."

I walk into Mom's hospital room. She smiles when she sees me and asks, "Where am I?"

"You're in the hospital, Mom. You broke your arm."

"I did?"

Sometimes a poor memory is an advantage. Then, Mom asks me six more times, "Where am I?"

Mom is scheduled to be discharged after two days. I sit with her while the nurses gather up her things. There are no slacks because Mom had soiled them, so the nurses put on a hospital gown and a cotton robe which we can return later. There is no cast on her arm. The doctor puts on an immobilizer after Mom has a shot of Demerol. The immobilizer is like a heavy corset around the waist, upper arm and wrist to keep her arm still. It has Velcro closings. I know that spells trouble.

I take Mom back to "Ruby's Place." The residents are happy to see her and several of them say, "I missed you." Mom is still groggy and we put her in bed. She falls sound asleep.

Ruby says, "We'll watch her closely and call you if there is any change." I go to the drug store to get Mom's prescription filled (Tylenol with codeine). When I come back in about 15 minutes, Mom says, "They say I was in the hospital. Why didn't anybody tell me I was in the hospital? Everybody knew but me." I was amazed that she remembered their comments.

A few days go by and Ruby calls, "Your Mom took off the immobilizer. I took her to the emergency room. The orthopedic surgeon says she'll have to have surgery. He took x-rays and the bones are not healing correctly." I ask if Mom's doctor has seen her. "No, I made an appointment with him tomorrow at 9:45 A.M. I'll take her. I know you had an appointment with him for Thursday, but I don't think we should wait. Her arm doesn't look good."

"Thanks for the offer, Ruby, but I'll be there and take her to the doctor."

I leave at 7 A.M. for the two hour ride. Ruby has Mom up and dressed and she has eaten breakfast when I pick her up at 9. Mom looks at me and says, "Who are you?"

I say, "I'm Jennie."

"Are you my sister?" Mom has a sister named Jennie whom she hasn't mentioned in years. I am not sure if Mom is talking about her sister or about me whom she calls "Sister."

"I'm your daughter. You call me Sister." My eyes tear up. I thought it is important that I take her to the doctor. I thought it might comfort her. Anyone could have taken her.

The doctor says, "I'm sorry the immobilizer didn't work. I wanted to avoid surgery because of her age and all. He gives me a knowing look. He continues, "You'll have to take her to the hospital for lab tests. I'll do the EKG here." He looks at Mom. "You must be going dancing with your nails all painted." Mom grins, "You bet," she says, "You want to dance?'

Some doctors know how to relate to elderly patients. This doctor uses warmth and humor and "straight talk" about the condition. Mom trusts him and says, "Anything you say, Doc" when he tells her about the surgery to install a steel rod in her arm. He gives her a side-by-side hug.

The doctor looks at me and says, "The surgery will be Friday morning. Have her at the hospital around 6:30 A.M." Ruby says she would come in at 5 A.M. and give Mom a shampoo and shower and have her ready at 6.

I call my brother to tell him about the surgery and to ask him if he could come and help me out. I tell him about the slumber party which was to begin on Saturday morning. I tell him that I will be with Mom all day Friday (the day of the surgery) and I could take turns with him being with Mom on Saturday and Sunday. He says, "I'll call you back."

The phone rings an hour later. My brother says, "I think you should get a nurse for Mom. It's in her best interest."

I ask, "What's the bottom line? Are you coming?"

He says, "No."

Damn him. It's his mother too. He never helps out. I don't know what to do about the weekend. I decide to cancel it. Dick says, "I'll sit with your Mom on Saturday and Sunday." Laurie, our daughter, says she will sit with her too. Ruby says she will help. My neighbor across the street at the lake home says, "Call me if I can do anything." Thank God, I am not alone. I don't cancel the slumber party. Dick feels strongly that I need some respite.

I take Mom to the hospital for a urinalysis and blood tests. She doesn't like the tests and asks constantly, "Where am I?" and "Why am I here?" The next day, Ruby calls to say, "The hospital can't find her lab tests which they took yesterday and they forgot to put a yellow band on her arm with her blood type. I'll take her back this afternoon. I told the hospital that you drove four hours round trip just for those lab tests."

This is one of those times I just want to scream. Mom is going to have to go through the whole procedure again because of somebody's incompetence. I'm sure they don't realize the effort it takes just to dress Mom, not to mention preparing her for the needle and just getting her there. She can become very hostile. I wouldn't blame her this time.

"Thanks again, Ruby."

Mom is sleepy-eyed but showered and dressed at 6 A.M., the day of the surgery. She keeps looking at me as we drive to the hospital.

"Where are we going?"

"To the hospital to get your arm fixed."

"My arm's okay."

"Your arm is broken, Mom, and needs fixing."

"Okay."

This dialogue is repeated many times before we reach the hospital. I remain calm each time she asks. I have learned to be patient. This is something Mom has taught me.

I am able to get a parking space near the front entrance. I know I can't drop her off to park because I don't know what she would do in the few minutes while I park the car.

We get halfway to the front door. She says, "I don't think I can make it." She slumps forward slightly and I hold her for a minute. Then, we go in and get a wheelchair and register her for surgery.

The small room is cold. She keeps saying, "I'm cold, I'm cold." The nurse takes her coat and top off and goes to get some papers. Mom repeats, "I'm cold." I cover her up with a blanket. Another nurse finally brings her a heated blanket. Mom says, "That's good" and falls asleep.

In a few minutes, another nurse comes in and pulls the covers back. Mom rises up to a sitting position (broken arm and all) and says, "What the hell do you think you're doing?"

"I'm going to put these surgical stockings on you and give you a shot for surgery."

Mom says, "Oh" and falls back asleep. A half hour later, Mom is put on a wheeled cart and taken to surgery.

I stop off at the sanctuary, a small chapel in the hospital. I kneel down to pray that she suffer little and that she endure this ordeal so as to see better days free of pain. Then, I remember, she doesn't feel pain. My eyes are moist. The thought of opening up her frail, thin arm and putting a steel rod in it is too gruesome to think about. Instead, I think about how we will care for her after the surgery. She probably will be disoriented like the last surgery two years ago.

My prayers are answered. The surgery goes well. Mom is very disoriented for about a week. Then she is fine, but that week was awful. She is what they call a non-compliant patient. She is irritable and lashes out at everyone. She feels no pain. Her arm heals just fine.

I had the slumber party, but I arrived after the guests on Saturday because I went to the hospital early in the morning. I left the door open with a note. I start out totally exhausted. I have not slept well for two nights. I spent all day Friday with Mom. I went back early Saturday morning until Dick arrived. Bless his heart, as Mom used to say. I am renewed by old friends, laughter and happy times. I don't use any of the gourmet recipes. We didn't miss them.

19

The Itch

Brother of Ophir
Bright Adieu
Honor, the shortest route
To you.

—Emily Dickinson, 1880

Ruby's voice is low and deliberate. "Hello, Jennie, this is Ruby."

"Hi, Ruby."

Jennie, your Mom has a rash and it's evidently very itchy. I think she should see a doctor."

"Okay, I'll call her doctor and make an appointment. I'll call you back with the day and time."

"Thanks, Jennie."

I make an appointment and call Ruby. For the next few days before the appointment, I have nightmares about bugs crawling all over Mom and her intense scratching. I am always glad to wake up to end the terror.

The doctor says her rash (which is on her arms) is due to dry skin. He said it is common to the elderly. We can't blame it on the AD. The doctor gives me a prescription for a salve to rub on her arms. A few weeks later, Ruby calls and we talk about the itch. Now, Mom has a rash on her chest and her buttocks in addition to her arms. I take her back to the doctor. He wraps some gauze around her arms and then, puts on a covering which looks like a long glove. He says it might heal better. He decides to write a prescription for prednisone and another salve.

There is some improvement for a month. Then Mom starts scratching again. This time she scratches her legs, buttocks, chest, arms and hands. She scratches until there is blood. I make an appointment to take her to a dermatologist whom Ruby recommended.

I arrive at 9 A.M. to pick up Mom. Ruby says she will go with us because she has errands to do near the doctor's office. Ruby suggests that Mom go "potty" before the trip. Ruby has Mom on a toileting schedule to help prevent accidents. We go to the bathroom. Mom shouts at me, "Get out." Ruby starts to pull down Mom's slacks and diaper. Mom becomes very angry and shouts at Ruby, "You're mean. You don't know what you're doing. Get away. Get away."

Ruby asks Mom calmly, "Who are you talking to?"

Mom answers, "You."

I remember the times when I would try to help Mom and she would scream at me. I remember how I would become defensive at first and respond to her words. Later, I learned to simply forget my feelings and attempt to calm her with soothing words or some distraction. Maybe these outbursts are the only way Mom has now to express her frustration about being helped to go "potty." After all, she was a college-educated woman, and a person with a quick wit and a keen mind who never lacked for words to express her thoughts. I finally have learned that it's not Mom who is screaming. It is the Alzheimer's in her brain which is screaming. She is no longer responsible. She has lost herself. Ruby and I know this and accept Mom just "as is."

I help Mom put on her coat. She starts to hit me when I try to put on her hat. I wait a bit. When I open the door which leads to the parking lot, Mom says, "It's cold." I put on her hat. Sometimes, it helps to wait. It sometimes avoids her increased agitation. Confrontation doesn't work.

She backs into the seat slowly. I put her legs in the car and start to put on her seat belt. She gives me an icy stare and fists her hands. I step back and say, "I love you" and hug her. At the same time, I hook her seat belt. You learn.

I follow Ruby's car and occasionally glance at Mom. Her wool knit hat keeps creeping forward and it is annoying her. I reach over to push it back and I see the same icy stare and fisting. I wait and then reach for the hat from the back of her head. This is okay and she settles down.

There is construction around the doctor's office and parking is rerouted. This means about a two-block walk to the office. I park and look for Ruby. She is nowhere in sight. I wait for five minutes and then ask Mom to get out of the car, please. She gets out and is immediately assaulted by the winter winds of January. She whines, "I can't walk. It's too cold. My legs are breaking." We turn around and head back to the car. It seems like an eternity before we get back. She keeps saying, "I can't. I can't." I say, "Mom, don't say I can't, say I will try." There is a quick glimmer of recognition. Then, she goes vacant in the eyes again. She's dying with open eyes. I keep saying, "It's nice and warm in the car. Keep going. We'll be there soon."

When we reach the car door, she refuses to get in. At times like this, I wonder what her fear is and try to overcome it. "Let's get in where it's warm and we can go back to Ruby's Place later." She responds and backs into the seat. I swing her legs in and we are off. Now what?

I decide to drive to the hospital which is connected to the doctor's office building. I get out of the car after parking in front of the hospital. I lock her in the car with her seat belt on and run to the hospital entrance and take a wheelchair out to the car. I am determined to get her to the dermatologist to get rid of the itching. I would climb a mountain to accomplish that goal. I am too close to give up now. I don't want to start all over again another day.

Mom finally agrees to get out of the car. She whines all the way to the hospital door. "It's going to be okay. We're almost there," I say softly. Comforting words seem to work better than ignoring or rejecting complaints.

I don't know the name of the dermatologist or his office number. Ruby did, but she isn't here. Fortunately, the dermatologist is the only one in town and a kind lady at the front desk offers to watch Mom while I move the car from the hospital entrance. This lady gives me directions through the hospital and says, "Just bring the wheelchair back here and I'll watch her while you get your car." I say, "Bless you." Some others might have said that the wheelchair is only for hospital patients. She didn't. If she had, I was prepared to make my case. There was no way I could get Mom to the doctor's office without a wheelchair.

When we finally reach the doctor's office, she refuses to take off her hat and coat. I just unbutton her coat and proceed to fill out forms. Ruby left a message that she missed us in the parking lot and she went on her errands.

The doctor comes out and introduces himself. This is different. Usually, we are ushered into a room by someone else. He even pushes the wheelchair into his examining room. I tell him that Mom doesn't want to take off her coat and hat, but I will try again. He says, "Let me see what I can do without upsetting her." What a relief! Here is someone who understands.

He pushes her sleeves back and she yells, "Stop it. Don't let him do that." The doctor talks soothingly and continues his examination. I am his backup saying, "He's trying to help you with your itch. It's okay." She continues to yell at the doctor. He says there are three possibilities for the rash. He writes a prescription for prednisone and asks me to call him in three weeks about her progress.

I pay the bill and push the wheelchair through the doctor's building into the hospital. When we get to the reception desk, that sweet lady is there. She smiles warmly at Mom who smiles back. She looks at me and says, "Go ahead, we are going to chat for awhile," and she looks at Mom. This lady has made all things possible today. I thank her profusely. I drive the car to the entrance and there is the lady and Mom waiting. I am so overcome with gratitude that tears fill my eyes. There are many good people in the world.

I ponder many thoughts as I drive while Mom dozes off. She is beginning to take naps in the middle of the day. I wonder why people don't make it easier for a drop-off at hospitals and doctor's offices. Sure, there is the emergency entrance but that's for emergencies. I wonder why there aren't more flexible and caring people to help in little ways to make a big difference. Maybe, people need to know more about Alzheimer's disease, not just those who have it and those who are caregivers. Mostly, I agree with the Alzheimer's Association whose vision is a world without Alzheimer's.

20

Broken Wrist

"Faith" is a fine invention
When Gentlemen can see-
But Microscopes are prudent
In an Emergency.

—Emily Dickinson, 1860

The telephone rings. I run to reach it before the fourth ring when the message recorder starts.

"Jennie, Ruby here. Your mother's wrist was black and blue this morning and the girls (on duty) decided she should have it x-rayed and we took her to the emergency room.

How is she, Ruby?"

"Well, the x-rays showed no broken bones and they recommended we take her to her regular doctor. We called him and he couldn't take her right away so we scheduled her with a new doctor in the same office. The new doctor said your Mom has a hairline fracture and he is going to use a splint rather than a cast on her".

"Is there anything we need to do?"

"She has to go back to the doctor on Monday. I can take her if you want me to. The appointment is 2 P.M.

"I'll take her. Thanks, Ruby."

The doctor says, "Let's get a new x-ray and see if the fracture is healing." Mom has the x-ray and we go back to the examining room to wait for the doctor. Every two to three minutes, Mom says, "Let's go." I say, "We're waiting for the doctor. He wants to see you." She is clearly getting agitated by the wait.

Finally the doctor comes in and says, "It's healing nicely."

I ask, "How long will the splint be on her arm?"

"It will be just a little longer. Then, we'll consider physical therapy to bring back the range of motion in her wrist."

I ask, "May I see the x-ray?"

He takes the x-ray and puts it in front of the light. He says, "Actually, I can't see a fracture here. A radiologist would have to look at it."

I tell him that a radiologist has already seen it at the hospital and said that there were no fractures."

The doctor says, "Really."

Here's Mom wearing a splint and about to start on a physical therapy regimen for a fracture which isn't there. I say, "Let's get out of here."

I make an appointment with Mom's regular doctor. I tell him that I am not convinced that she has a fracture. He reads the records and the x-rays and takes off Mom's splint. He is surprised and dismayed that Mom's rash is worse. He immediately leaves the room and comes back with sterile gloves, some salve, and some cotton covering for her arms and hands. He doesn't ask the nurse to do it but he proceeds to tenderly rub her arms and hands with the salve and then covers them with a cotton sleeve.

We discuss Mom's medication. The medicine for the itching is making her drowsy all day. I tell the doctor that she cannot stay awake for more than five minutes. He changes her day and night medications for a few days.

The doctor leaves the room for about ten minutes. Mom's chart is left open on the shelf. I glance at it. The other doctor made an entry which said that he doubted if a fracture existed. Yet, she was wearing that splint over her rash. Another entry in the chart by her regular doctor said, "She's a sweetheart." Mom is lucky to have a doctor who cares so much.

Her regular doctor gives Mom a hug and a chocolate kiss wrapped in foil. Mom looks at the object in her hand. When I unwrap it and tell her its candy, she grins and pops it in her mouth. I remember my children getting lollipops from their pediatrician.

Things settle down after that. Mom's rash clears up and she enjoys two wonderful years at Ruby's Place. As her condition deteriorates, she is moved into the Alzheimer's unit adjoining the CBRF. Ruby would have kept Mom, but the licensing person for the county says she can no longer stay there. Camelot is over. The unit next door has more staff and only eight residents. Of course, the cost is higher. Mom ran out of her money several years ago. I'm sure that people don't realize the high costs of Alzheimer's care. We certainly didn't have a clue.

The residents in the AD unit need a lot of care. Over a few months, we see quite a bit of staff turnover. It must be very difficult to care for eight people, all of whom have advanced Alzheimer's disease. In fact, all of them are in the final stage of the disease.

21

Cancel Everything

Taking up the fair ideal,
Just to cast her down
When a fracture-we discover-
Or a splinter crown-

—(Excerpt from "Taking up the fair ideal")
Emily Dickinson, 1862

It has been a long cold winter with gray skies, lots of snow and very few sunny days. Dick and I decide to go to Branson, Missouri, the country music haven, for a few days. I spend several weeks researching accommodations and we make reservations at a lodge on a lake. The Branson Chamber of Commerce sent me a schedule of the music shows and I call and make a few reservations.

It's going to be good to have a respite. Mom has made a good adjustment to the Alzheimer's home. We are satisfied with her care. She is always clean and appears happy. Though sleepy a lot of the time, she can be aroused easily. She falls back asleep, however, into a deep slumber almost immediately.

The staff also has Mom on a toileting schedule. An aide puts her on the toilet several times a day. She wears an adult diaper with an elastic waistband because it's easier to pull on and off. At night, she wears the diaper with the Velcro closures. Her diapers are changed twice during the night to prevent odors and skin problems. It works. There is never an unpleasant odor in her room or in the unit.

It is one week before we are to leave for Missouri. I check all of Mom's papers to make sure they are in order. While glancing at her Durable Power of Attorney for Health Care form, I notice that it becomes effective only when two doctors document in a written form that Mom is incapacitated. This is the standard form for the state. I call her doctor and request the documentation.

When I call, I find out that Mom is on her way to the doctor. I hang up and call the AD unit because I'm concerned that something is wrong. The Director says, "We were just going to call you. Your Mom is complaining about her knee and she refuses to stand or walk. We thought we had better check it out."

I say, "While you're there, would you remind the doctor about written documentation of Mom's incapacity?"

"Sure, what do you need?"

"I need a statement in writing from two doctors that Mom is incompetent. His associate has seen Mom in the past."

"Okay, I'll call you when I get back."

After several hours go by, the Director of the AD unit calls me.

"Jennie, your Mom has a broken hip. She's scheduled to have surgery tomorrow."

What time?"

"It will be first thing in the morning."

Mom is going to have major surgery again. In the last few years, Mom has had a complete hysterectomy, a steel rod placed in her upper arm, a screw placed in her elbow, and now a metal ball will be put in her hip. She is a bionic senior citizen. I'm just thankful that she doesn't experience much pain.

The surgery is scheduled for Saturday morning at 8 A.M., the day before Easter. I was going to have the whole family over for dinner on Sunday.

I ask Dick, "What are we going to do about Easter and Missouri?"

Dick says simply, "Cancel everything." I know that Dick is disappointed because we haven't been on a vacation for many years.

I call and cancel the Missouri reservations for the lodge and shows. I sit down and weep. I am feeling like a puppet on a string being yanked up and down by someone who doesn't recognize me or anyone else. Mom has had total control of my life in her last 10 years of Alzheimer's disease. I have been called upon to drop everything for a loved one occasionally, but 10 years is a long time for her complete care to hover over me.

I want to call my brother and yell, "Get over here, you horse's ass and help out. It's your turn." But I've called him several times for help and he has never come through. He is too self-involved. He was never present for any of her operations. I am writing him off now. I won't even frustrate myself further by calling him.

I thank God for Dick. He is more like a son to Mom, and also a great support to me.

According to Safford in *Caring For the Mentally Impaired Elderly*:

Caring for a mentally impaired person has been compared to a funeral without end, but it is much more painful than a funeral. A funeral provides the opportunity to release our emotions in the company of family and friends, and it lasts only a few hours. But the period of caring for the mentally impaired lasts much longer and there's limited support from family and friends. It is much, much worse than a funeral. It is bereavement with no end in sight.

I call our family and tell them the news about the surgery. They are all in Illinois and we are in Wisconsin. They all decide to drive four hours to see Mom and spend Easter with Dick and me. I weep again with gratitude. We are so lucky to have supportive and caring children and grandchildren. We don't have to cancel everything after all.

22

Hospital Days

Presentiment-is that long Shadow-on the Lawn-
Indicative that Suns go down-

The notice to the startled Grass
That Darkness-is about to pass-

—Emily Dickinson, 1863

Dick and I and our daughter, Laurie, and her children leave for the trip to the hospital on the day before the surgery. We drive straight to the hospital. Mom is sound asleep. The world of Alzheimer's has some advantages. Without memory, she has no fear of coming events. She doesn't worry. She is suspended in the now of life which lasts only seconds. The Buddhists believe in the power of now, but somehow I don't think this state is what they mean. It's difficult to imagine this kind of existence. At any rate, she has no pre-surgery jitters.

The nurse at the nursing station says, "I'm glad you came. I was going to call you. We need you to sign for her surgery". "Here are the papers. Just sign here." She puts another paper down and says, "Sign here."

All I can think about is that I need documentation from two doctors for the Power of Attorney for Health Care and I still don't have it. I do have a Durable Power of Attorney which would cover everything, but if there is a question about health care, I don't want to leave any stone unturned.

I sleep fitfully that night. I have the pre-surgery jitters. Without the documentation for incapacity, I dream that a health care decision needs to be made and they keep hammering Mom with questions and she just looks at them with vacant eyes and an occasional smile. They don't know she is incompetent without paperwork! What a nightmare!

It is still dark when Dick and I leave for the hospital on the morning of the surgery. After an hour, the doctor comes in. I ask him about the documentation requested earlier.

"I'll have it typed Monday," he says.

I ask, "What about the surgery?"

"Don't worry. This is an emergency. I'm assuming that if she stops breathing, we won't start with a respirator. She'll probably be fine and they'll get her up and walking the day after surgery."

"She'll walk the day after surgery?"

"Yes, it's better that way."

I have to admit I am a little stunned by the reference to no respirator. I do agree though. Mom has been the real puppet in all of this. She trustfully has followed anyone's lead. She is a precious jewel full of unconditional love, a real inspiration at times and a real frustration at times.

Her surgeon walks in briskly wearing his green cotton pants and slipover shirt with a small matching head cover. He looks very young and has an athletic build. For a moment, I imagine that they called the new guy in a practice to do surgery on a Saturday at the last minute. As he talks, I forget about his youthful appearance. He appears confident, competent, and willing to answer our questions. He doesn't mention the respirator.

"Doctor, would you be willing to sign documentation of her incapacity?" I ask.

"Usually that is done by her family doctor," he replies.

"Yes, he has agreed, but I need two doctors."

"Don't worry. We'll take care of it."

Mom is wheeled into surgery. I do not have the two signatures.

We are joined by Jeff in the waiting room for families of surgical patients. There is no coffee or volunteer because it is Saturday. There are some pamphlets and magazines. I read about cancer, dying, heart disease, funeral preparations, and other heavy issues. There are no funny books here.

Suddenly, her family doctor, a robust German-American, enters the room. "Everything's fine. We wanted to use a spinal but we had to give her a general anesthetic." He proceeds to explain the total hip replacement. I think he exemplifies a great doctor. He is caring. He listens and acts on what he hears. He also teaches as he talks. He tells us to go and have some coffee because Mom will be in the recovery room for at least an hour.

We go to the hospital coffee shop and have a wonderful breakfast prepared by a volunteer. Jeff, Dick, and I have large omelets, hash browns, and coffee. The volunteer says, "You buy one cup and you can have free coffee all day." Jeff says, "It's worth the two hour trip just to have breakfast here." Jeff is making light of his contribution of support, but he always comes through when we need him. This is true with all of our children. If there ever was a test for unconditional love, Alzheimer's is it. Our children pass it with flying colors.

We all feel a tremendous relief that we didn't have to deal with the respirator question, but then, we feel bad for all that Mom has endured and will still endure as she faces her recovery.

Laurie, our daughter, and her three children arrive when Mom is in her room. The two older grandchildren, Ryan and Jamie, look a little startled when they see their great-grandmother primarily because she doesn't have her false teeth in her mouth. Her lips look like they have been swallowed. Ryan and Jamie are especially quiet. Little Mollie, 10 months old, smiles and lightens the moment with her, "Ba-ba-ba." She, like her Great-grandmother, lives in the now, but she is moving in a positive direction. Poor Mom. She is going backwards.

We stay awhile until the nurse says, "She's doing fine and will probably sleep the rest of the day."

We all leave with a sense of renewal, that Easter feeling.

23

Post-op

"Hope" is a thing with feathers-
That perches in the soul-
And sings the tune without the words-
And never stops—at all-

And sweetest-in the Gale-is heard-
And sore must be the storm-
That could abash the little Bird
That kept so many warm-

I've heard it in the chillest land-
And on the strangest Sea-
Yet never, in Extremity,
It asked a crumb of Me.

—Emily Dickinson, 1861

Our son, Scott, his wife, and three children meet us at the hospital on Easter Sunday. No one goes to church. We have a special pilgrimage at the hospital.

Mom is still sleeping even though three preschoolers with boundless energy surround her. They are dressed in Easter clothes (meant for church services) and are still elated by the visit from the Easter bunny, all except Kristin, our granddaughter. She leans against the wall and is very quiet. She glances up at great-gramma every few minutes. I put my arm around her and we share a special moment.

We stay as long as we think the hospital patients can tolerate the youthful exuberance of our grandchildren. Mom sleeps the whole time. I mention to the nurse that Mom's doctor said you would get her up today. The nurse says, "She's still too drowsy. Maybe we will try tomorrow."

We go back to our home and have Easter dinner. I have to admit that I get very sentimental for a moment. I am so overwhelmed with the support from our children that I say (with a tremulous voice and teary eyes), "Dad (Dick) and I are so grateful to have you here. We didn't ask you to come. I just hope your children are as supportive of you as you are of Dad and me." Scott says, "They'd better." We all have a hearty laugh. Scott always knows how to lighten a tense moment. I look at him and think, "He is a great father, just like his Dad."

The afternoon is filled with children happily playing, sports on the TV, and conversations to catch up on each other's lives. Soon, it is time for our children to head back home on the two hour ride. They leave and the quietness is very loud.

Dick and I go back to the hospital. Mom is still asleep. I comb her hair and hug her. I tell her I love her. It is all I can do for her. Dick and I spend Monday and Tuesday with her. She wakes up very little. She still isn't walking.

On Wednesday, I ask the doctor about her sleeping all the time. He says he will change her medication from Tylenol with codeine to just Tylenol. He says that she is anemic and he orders two pints of blood. She still isn't walking.

The physical therapist comes in and throws back the covers of Mom's bed and raises and bends Mom's right leg three times. Then, she puts Mom in a wheelchair. She is still asleep. The therapist tells me that her own mother has Alzheimer's and she put her mother in a nursing home in northern Wisconsin and left her there. She says, "I just couldn't deal with it." She leaves. But, for most of us caregivers, a nursing home means frequent visits, decision-making, and participation in care conferences, occasional outings if possible, and stacks of insurance forms, crisis management for illnesses or accidents, and a drain on the money supply. The caregiving is not ended. It is just shared. This sharing can be a Godsend.

I don't judge the therapist for her decision to separate herself from her mother who has Alzheimer's. I don't know what else she may be dealing with. Unless we walk in her shoes...

Mom is still not walking. I go to the nursing station and ask to see Mom's chart. A pretty young nurse says, I'll call Discharge Planning and see if it is all right." I remind the nurse that I have a Durable Power of Attorney.

"Discharge Planning says you can't see the chart until you have two doctor's signatures."

"But, I have a Durable Power of Attorney."

She says, "You can't have the chart unless you have the two signatures." The young nurse smiles sweetly and says, "I'm following orders."

I feel like bopping her over the head. I can feel my rage as blood rushes to my head. My face is flushed. I sit quietly for the storm to subside. This seems to work for me. I am not a yeller. I say to Dick, "Isn't it funny (peculiar) that I was able to sign for her surgery, but I can't see her chart?"

I've known some medical bureaucrats who overlook patient's needs in the name of "I'm just doing my job" or I'm just following orders." They are self-appointed bureaucrats in my experience. They could seek a solution that doesn't break the rules but attends to the patients needs. I do believe in following rules but there is a way to present them and to overcome them if not appropriate. In this case, Discharge Planning could contact the doctor about the documentation.

I tell Mom's doctor about the chart incident. He shakes his head and hands me the letters of documentation. At last! One letter states:

> Cleo has been a patient in our clinic for several years. I have been observing her through three major surgeries: hysterectomy, fractured humerus, and also a fractured hip. Cleo is a very lovely lady, but at 92, she has had advanced Alzheimer's disease for many years. She is completely detached from the present and certainly incapable to make her own decisions. She does not know, nor understand her environment. She has true Alzheimer's disease and needs a guardian for decision-making.

The other letter stated:

> This 92 year old female has Alzheimer's and dementia. She is unable to care for herself and make necessary decisions of living. I have seen her on a few occasions for her wrist fracture.

Mom's doctor says he is ordering Mom another pint of blood for her anemia. This should help her be more alert. He says he is preparing for Mom's discharge soon. I say, "I hope she will be able to go back to the Alzheimer's unit."

Dick and I receive word that an old friend has died of cancer. We drive two hours for the funeral and return Friday to the hospital. Mom is sleeping. The physical therapist has managed to get her to walk a few steps but she has her eyes closed at the time. I wonder, "Is she dying or is she still coming out of the anesthesia?" I've heard that the effects of anesthesia sometimes last longer on the elderly.

The Director of the Alzheimer's unit stops in to visit Mom. Then the Discharge Planner comes in. We talk about plans after hospitalization. The physical therapist comes in. She says Mom needs two people to assist her to walk and that she only walked a few steps the day before. She and an associate get Mom out of bed (still sleeping) and lift her for about seven steps and seat her in the wheelchair. I don't call that walking. Maybe, it's a new form of sleep-walking.

The Director says, "I don't see how we can take her back to the Alzheimer's unit since she needs two people to assist her. We have people who go out the door and someone has to be available to go after them." I have trouble with this because many of the people in the AD unit occasionally need two people. "Ruby has taken people back in her unit after hip surgery," I say pleadingly.

"I know," she says, "But I don't think it is fair to the other residents if she comes back requiring two people. I hope you understand, Jennie." I know that Ruby would take her back if she could but her licensing doesn't allow it. Ruby thinks of her residents as family and, certainly, if a family member has surgery, you take care of them. You don't kick them out. This Director sees it differently.

I realize it is a lost cause. The Director of the AD unit stands firm. Mom may not return. The Discharge Planner realizes it too and says, "She could go to a nursing home for the short-term and then, if she improved to where she needed only one person for walking, she could go back to the AD unit."

"Which nursing home are you talking about?" I ask with my voice quivering.

"There are three in the area which have openings."

"Which do you recommend?"

"I can't recommend. I can only tell you what's available. Perhaps, you could visit them today and call me before 2:30 P.M. because the doctor will probably discharge her tomorrow." I have 24 hours for this major decision. At least, I am able to make the decision. The documentation of incompetence is now in her chart.

I sob openly. Mom has to move again. When will this nightmare end? The Director holds my hand. Ruby would have hugged me. I miss Ruby.

The Discharge Planner gives me the names of the three nursing homes. She suggests that we visit unannounced to see the "real" picture. I hate the responsibility of entrusting Mom to the care of others when she can't advocate for herself.

24

Finding a Nursing Home Again

There is a Languor of the Life
More imminent than Pain-
"Tis Pain's Successor-When the Soul
Has suffered all it can-

A Drowsiness-diffuses-
A Dimness like a Fog
Envelopes Consciousness-
As Mists-obliterate a Crag.

—(Excerpt from "There is a Languor of the Life")
Emily Dickinson, 1862

We have three nursing home options. One home gives bonuses just to get people to work there. Several people have told us horror stories about it. We decide to do a "drive-by" and not visit. The second home is a very large complex serving 500 people. We walk down several corridors. There is no one in the corridors. All of the residents are in their rooms. No one is at the reception desk. We wander around. We don't see any staff. Finally, someone walking out of a door says, "May I help you?"

"We're looking for Social Services."

"Go down this corridor and turn left. Go to the elevator and get off at the second floor."

We go down the corridor. Everything is very clean. There is a sitting room on the left. No one is sitting in it. We go to the second floor. The Social Services area is unoccupied. Then, a very heavy-set woman shuffles past us. We ask, "Could you tell us where we could find someone from Social Services?"

"It's over there. Do you have an appointment?" she asks.

"No, but my Mom is in a local hospital and will be discharged tomorrow. We were asked to visit today."

"That's unusual. Usually, the hospital gives us more lead time. I don't even know if there is an opening."

"The Discharge Planner said there was an opening."

"Even if there is an opening, I don't know if your mother would be eligible," she replies in a gruff voice.

"Where would the Alzheimer's unit be?"

She says, with obvious impatience, "They're on the third floor. We don't like people visiting without a staff member. There may not be an opening."

I look at her eye-to-eye and say, "Do you know what it's like to have a mother with Alzheimer's disease? Do you know what it's like to have three choices of nursing homes? Do you know what it's like when two of the three choices are not good? Do you know what it's like to have someone tell you, not once but three times, that you don't know if there is an opening when I told you the hospital checked and there was an opening?"

I look at her name tag and am shocked to see, in small letters under her name, *Social Services*. She has acted as if no one is available from Social Services. There must be an extreme shortage of staff for this insensitive woman to be employed. Dick says, "Let's go."

I say, "My Mother will not be coming here. This is a warehouse. Residents are stored in their rooms and there is no apparent socialization. All I can say is God bless these residents." Dick and I leave quickly. In this large complex, we see only one staff member whose function is questionable in our eyes. Each resident is in their room just sitting or sleeping. No wonder we were advised to visit unannounced.

We drive to our last choice. We feel a sense of desperation. We dare not think about what we would do if this home is not satisfactory. We park and enter the side door which immediately sets off an alarm. We have entered the emergency door. It is no longer an unannounced visit. A smiling and attractive young lady turns off the alarm and says, "That's okay," to our apologies. She explains that the alarm is for residents who wander out the door.

We walk to the nursing station and are greeted warmly by a young lady who introduces herself as Tina. She says that a person from discharge planning from the hospital has called to say we might be visiting. She asks if we would like a tour. She introduces us to the residents and staff alike. She calls the residents by name and talks to them, not about them. We have questions about physical therapy. She says, "The therapists are eating lunch but they won't mind."

We talk with the physical and occupational therapists. They seem lighthearted and in good spirits. They ask questions about Mom's functioning. They say they will get her moving about. It seems like a positive energy is present in this nursing home.

We take a tour of the facility and ask many questions. We are satisfied with the answers. Tina apologizes for the construction which is going on. New wallpaper has to be put on the hall walls and in the dining room. Other rooms are being renovated. Little does she know that we are happy that improvements are being implemented. It makes the place seem more vital and alive, not static. We talk with several of the residents who think of the home as their home and the staff as extended family.

We feel relieved. This nursing home is small. It is a little larger than the CBRF but not anything like the warehouse we just visited. The staff is caring and welcomes family members to visit at any time. They have lots of activities. Local music and dancing groups perform regularly. While we were there, a local farmer brought in two baby calves. The residents loved them. They held them and fed them from a bottle. The place was alive with life. There were no unpleasant smells. This home is also close to our lake house. The other two nursing homes were in another small town nearby.

We sign the pre-admission papers; give Tina copies of the Durable Power of Attorney, the Durable Power of Attorney for Health Care, Mom's Living Will, and Medicare and supplementary insurance cards. Tina gives us some information about rehabilitation and tells us that we will have to fill out about 15 pages upon admittance. She asks, "Do you have any other questions?" We don't, so Tina turns off the alarm for a minute so we can exit the same door we came in because it is closer.

We sit in the car and agree that this is the best of the three choices. The other two weren't a consideration. We feel good about this home. This will be Mom's third move in three months. First, there was the move to the Alzheimer's unit, then to the hospital, and now to the nursing home. We are silent with our sadness.

25

The Visits

I dwell in Possibility-
A fairer House than Prose-
More numerous of Windows-
Superior-for Doors-

Of Chambers as the Cedars-
Impregnable of Eye-
And for an Everlasting Roof
The Gambrels of the Sky-

Of Visitors-the fairest-
For Occupation-this-
The spreading wide my narrow Hands
To gather Paradise-

—Emily Dickinson, 1862

    I sign in at the nursing home. Only two people have signed in as visitors since I was here yesterday. As I walk past the nursing station, the social worker says, "Hi, Jennie." I am surprised that she remembers my name. In general, I have always been Cleo's daughter or her representative depending on the situation. Here, I am a person in my own right. The physical therapist who works with Mom smiles a greeting. I appreciate a physical therapist (P.T.) who is in apparently good condition. I think it means they practice their beliefs. This P.T. is tall, slim, personable, and caring.

    I walk down the hall that's a little brighter today because the sun is finally shining after four cloudy days. As I look in each room, I find myself thinking that each person holds the ending of a life story. One gentleman is sitting in a wheelchair with his head resting on his shoulders watching TV. His expression never changes. He doesn't appear to move from this position. Another gentleman is sitting in a wheelchair but his head is leaning forward almost touching the lap tray. His eyes are closed and a long stream of mucus is falling from his nose on to the tray. At first, I am repulsed. Then, I walk in and wipe his nose with a tissue from his night stand. One's dignity is something we all share.

Mom's roommate approaches me. She is dressed in a pink sweatshirt, common attire for a nursing home because you can wear it day and night. "Did you and Cleo get along okay?"

"I haven't talked to her. She's always asleep," the roommate responds.

"Yes, Mom had surgery on her hip and she hasn't really come to."

"I think it's awful the way they force food in her when she's sleeping. It is downright mean."

"They're just trying to get her to eat," I say with mixed feelings. I am hoping and praying that the feeding is being done gently. I'm not sure how reliable her roommate is as an observer. I also know how frustrating it is to feed Mom when she clamps her gums shut and refuses to open them. She has refused to wear her dentures for some time now.

I find Mom sound asleep in her wheelchair. Her hair is combed (unlike in the hospital) and she has on a clean set of clothes. She doesn't stir.

"Hello, Cleo," I say as I take both of her hands in mine. She opens her eyes. She looks startled and blank and she quickly closes them. It's been a long time since we've had a real talk other than, "How are you?" and she says, "Pretty good" or "Not good." I'm never sure that she knows what she's saying even then.

Today, I sit for a half-hour and watch her sleep. She doesn't move her arms or legs. Her eyes occasionally flutter under the lids and her tongue moves sideways in her mouth. Her lips are slightly parted.

I go through the "Mom" routine again. Then I say, "Hello, Cleo." It is strange to me to call Mom by her first name. She still doesn't wake up. Once her eyebrows raise high and I think she's waking up, but her eyes never open.

I proceed to tell Mom all about her grandchildren and great-grandchildren, and anything else going on in the family. I only have these conversations with Mom when we are alone. Sometimes, people in a coma hear conversations. I don't want to leave any stone unturned. Intellectually, I know she is not mentally aware. She left her body a long time ago. Her body is now in a resting place, in a waiting room of sorts. She is waiting for her body to release her, it seems to me.

I slip out of her room and out of the nursing home and into the bright light of day where people are breathing fresh air and living freely. I feel a sense of renewal.

Mom seems at peace at the nursing home. I make a special dinner for Dick and we sit down to eat. The phone rings.

"Hello, this is Joan from the nursing home. Cleo just fell out of the wheelchair. I have checked her all over and she is fine. It is our policy to let the family know when something like this happens." I suggest that Mom have a restraint so that she doesn't fall again. The nurse says she will request a restraint order from the doctor.

Dick and I hurriedly finish dinner and drive to the nursing home. We are both numb with, "What's next?"

Mom is sitting in the wheelchair. She has a strap around her waist which is attached to the wheelchair. She is sound asleep. She does not respond to our greeting. Every few minutes, she leans forward as far as the strap will allow and hangs her head down.

The nurse who called us says, "She's doing okay. I called the doctor. He said the restraint is okay since you requested it and it is for her safety. We're having trouble getting her to eat. We puree her food. If there is the smallest lump, she spits it out. She ate a few spoons of jello and that's all."

I mention, "At the hospital, if she wouldn't eat, they would feed her with a syringe."

"Oh, we can't do that. There is a risk she could aspirate." I shudder to think of the many times I fed her at the hospital with the syringe at the nurse's request.

"Have you tried a baby-sized spoon?" I ask.

"No, that's a good idea," she says.

"Sometimes, she'll drink through a straw," I add.

Mom looks uncomfortable in her wheelchair. She pulls at her sweat pants until they are up to her knees. She, then, rocks back and forth.

"Are you okay, Mom?" I ask.

"No."

"Are you in pain?"

"Yes."

"What hurts?"

There is no response. Mom goes back to sleep with a frown on her face. I ring the bell for the nurse. I tell her, "She's very uncomfortable. I think she is ready to go to bed." The nurse asks us to step out. This request always makes me uncomfortable especially since we have been Mom's caregivers for ten years.

We wait in the hall. Dick twitches my cheek and smiles at me. I can't smile back. I am lost in my thoughts. I wonder how long she would have sat there if we had not come and summoned the nurse.

We say good-night to Mom, but she is already asleep. Her roommate says, "She's a mystery to herself."

"Well said," I add.

26

Dental Care

To fill a Gap
Insert the Thing that caused it-
Block it up
With other-and 'twill yawn the more-
You cannot solder an Abyss
With Air.

—Emily Dickinson, 1862

The nursing home assistant telephones me and asks if Mom has seen a dentist in the last year. She says, "All residents of nursing homes are required to have an annual dental report on file. If she has seen a dentist, we can request the report."

"No, she hasn't seen a dentist in years. She is supposed to wear dentures but has refused to wear them for the past eight months. Before that, she would hide them in plants, in the toilet, under the bed or mattress, just anywhere. We thought about taking her to the dentist, but I knew she wouldn't probably open her mouth for a checkup."

"We have to follow the rules. We have a dentist who comes to the nursing home. Would you like for me to schedule your Mom for a checkup?"

"Sure."

I wonder if Mom will open her mouth for the dentist. I remember when I took Mom to the dentist to get new dentures years ago; she gagged and gagged when the dentist put some white putty-like material in her mouth to make an impression. The dentist was very patient and finally got an impression for the dentures. That was a long time ago when she would cooperate.

Several weeks go by and the dentist calls me. She says that Mom has only one tooth in her mouth and it has a cavity. She says she had a very difficult time just looking in her mouth and, in her opinion, it would be impossible to fill the cavity. On the other hand, the cavity may cause her pain, so she recommends that either the tooth be pulled by an oral surgeon who would sedate her or else we could wait until the tooth caused Mom pain and then have it pulled.

We have more decisions. What would I want done if I was in Mom's shoes? Well, she doesn't appear to feel pain. On the other hand, the effects of the anesthesia from her last surgery lasted six months and she was still not the same as before the surgery. Also, her lower denture slips over the one tooth left in her mouth. If she ever lets us put the dentures back in, would the tooth be important? There is no way we could get another impression. She simply would not tolerate it.

I decide to delay the extraction of the tooth mainly because of my concerns over the sedation effects. The dentist says, "That will be fine."

After I hang up, I worry about the decision and almost call the dentist back to schedule the extraction. Then, I talk with Dick and we agree that we can always request the extraction later. Mom's dealing with a lot right now. She is sleeping about twenty hours a day. She is being fed pureed food. She can no longer walk and is spending her days in her wheelchair, frequently bent forward so far that her head almost touches her knees. If she isn't restrained by a belt, she will topple on the floor. She is incontinent. Her vision and hearing are poor. She refuses to wear her glasses, her hearing aids, and her dentures. Her speech is mostly gibberish and we strain to make sense of it. Her mind is gone. Now, it seems that her last tooth might have to go.

27

Emma

I'm Nobody! Who are you?
Are you—Nobody—too?
Then there's a pair of us!
Don't tell! They'd advertise—you know!

—Emily Dickinson, 1861
(Excerpt from "I'm Nobody! Who are you?")

Each time I go to the nursing home, if Mom is in her wheelchair, I push her around the halls. It is my way of saying. "Mom, there's more to life than your room." I tell her about the weather if we can't go outside. I tell her about the late-breaking news of the day. She either sleeps or lets out her rhythmic moan. These distinctive sounds remind the nurses of the sound of the morning dove. Some of them call her "The Morning Dove." The dove is a widespread inhabitant of Wisconsin. They are enduring, gracious and beautiful birds. I think it fits. Much later, I find out that the birds are "Mourning Doves" and not morning doves. It fits even better.

One day, a little old lady in a wheelchair inches along the hallway by herself. Tears are welled up in her eyes. She grabs me by the arm.

"Do you know where my room is?"

I reply, "No, I don't but I'm sure a nurse will come by soon and show you. I take a few steps forward and see that the names of the residents are on a placard outside of each room.

"Maybe I can help you. What is your name?"

"Emma."

She tells us her last name and Dick pushes Emma and I push Mom as we look at each placard for Emma's room. Emma has tears in her eyes, tears of joy. It's the small things that count. I remember the kind lady at the hospital who helped me.

Emma is happy. She is no longer lost. Everyone needs a sense of belonging. I feel sorry for Mom. She has been lost for some time.

The next day after breakfast, I go to see Mom. She isn't in her room. Her roommate says she is in the activity room. The staff said they are going to move Mom to a room closer to the therapy room today but her things are still in the old room.

There she is. She is sitting in the middle of the activity room surrounded by loud music and exercise directions with about 15 people responding to the activity in different ways. One man is in the back of the room and is not participating. He looks very sad. Another man is responding to the exercise with gusto following each new command. "Touch your hand. Stretch your arms high above your head." One lady is talking non-stop even though no one is listening. Some are asleep. Others are vaguely following along. The activities director goes from person to person and gently bats a balloon to each person. Mom wakes up and bats the balloon. She does a pretty good job hitting it each time. When the director leaves her, Mom falls asleep again.

Emma seems to have trouble batting the balloon. Then, I realize that she can't see very well. That's probably why she can't find her room. Then, Emma comes toward me and says, "Say, you're the one."

I jump because she startled me.

"I'm sorry. I scared you."

"That's okay."

"No, it's not good to be scared. I'm scared a lot."

"That doesn't feel good, does it?"

"No, they're always telling me what to do. I'm not as stupid as they think. I realize they have rules. I don't see well at all. I have this notebook and I'm trying to get all of my telephone numbers organized." Emma shows me a little spiral notebook.

"Do you have any children, Emma?"

"I have a daughter. She used to come and see me but the Lord gave her three little girls and she doesn't have time."

"Emma, you have time. Are you able to organize your numbers?"

"I try to but they are always interrupting me. I woke up early this morning before daylight to work on it but a nurse roaming the halls shut off my light and said, 'Go back to sleep.' It's very thwarting." Thwarting is an interesting word.

Then, Emma's face hardens and she clenches her dentures and says, "Can you sleep on command?"

"No, I can't, Emma" I respond. "By the way, Emma, where are you from?"

Emma brightens a bit and proceeds to tell me about herself. Then, the tears well up again when she says, "I don't belong here."

"Tell me about it, Emma."

This time, tears flow down her cheeks. She seems so little and helpless.

"It's a long story." Her chin trembles and the tears flow.

"I have time, Emma." Emma smiles.

Just then, an aide comes in and says, "Time to go, Emma."

Emma's right. They keep interrupting her. It is thwarting.

28

Autopsy Arrangements

All but Death, can be Adjusted-
Dynasties repaired-
Systems-settled in their Sockets-
Citadels—dissolved-

Wastes of Lives—renown with Colors
By Succeeding Springs-
Death—unto itself—Exception-
Is exempt from Change-

—Emily Dickinson, 1863

When I was studying neuropsychology, Mom was very interested in my text-books and tests. She and I believed that the brain sciences would one day unlock the many mysteries of the brain. Mom expressed an interest in how her own brain functioned. In the early days of her Alzheimer's disease, she would say, "I hope someday they'll find an answer to lost memories. I would like to donate my brain to science."

I started to investigate the possibility of an autopsy of Mom's brain tissue after her death. I wish that I had made arrangements years ago, not now that she is lying semiconscious and dehydrated in a nursing home. I feel an urgency to make arrangements as I remember her wish.

I call the national office of the Alzheimer's Association. I tell them that I think my Mom is dying and I need to know the procedure for a brain tissue autopsy. I am told that they will send me a pamphlet which will arrive in about three weeks. I ask if the pamphlet could be put in the mail today. I am told again that it will take three weeks. I ask if I can get information now. I am told that no one in the office knows anything about autopsy arrangements. I finally ask, "Who can I talk to about an autopsy?"

"Where does your mother live?" She asks.

"Wisconsin."

After a few minutes wait, she says, "A representative from the autopsy network lives in Eau Claire, Wisconsin. Here's her number." I am glad I am persistent.

I dial the number and get a recording which refers to another number. I call that number and the person who answered does not know anything about autopsies. She will have someone call me on Monday.

Early Monday morning, I receive a call and am referred to a local chapter of the Alzheimer's Association. A lady named Patty answers. I explain my need for autopsy procedures. She says she will find out and call me back. I wonder if this is going to be another dead end. I thought, no wonder there aren't more autopsies. No wonder we don't know the cause of Alzheimer's disease. It's a brain disease and research on the brain requires autopsies. In ten minutes, Patty calls me back. She tells me there are two locations possible, the Medical College in Milwaukee and the ALS clinic in Madison. Patty says she will get the details and call me tomorrow. Patty calls the next day. She gives me the details. I thank her. She says, "You don't need to do anymore than necessary when I can help. You've got enough going on. I'm happy to help." I wouldn't know Patty if I saw her, but we connected around an important issue. She's another one of those strangers who make a difference.

Later in the day, a representative from the Medical College calls me. She was referred by Patty. The representative explains the procedure. If I am interested, I can fill out the forms and return them to the Medical College. Then, upon Mom's death, I will have to send a telegram giving my permission for the brain autopsy. Mom's body will have to be transported within 12 hours for the brain tissue to be removed. Because of this time restraint, the nursing home has to be alerted to call me immediately. This instruction is to be placed in Mom's file at the nursing home. I gulp and ask, "How much does the autopsy cost?" I am told that my only cost will be the transportation of Mom's body to the Medical Center. I call a local funeral director and make preliminary arrangements for the transport so that, when the time comes, everyone will be prepared. Of course, we have no idea how much longer Mom will live.

This autopsy arrangement respects Mom's wishes and also means that Mom will continue in death as she did in life, to teach others.

29

The Advanced Stage

After great pain, a formal feeling comes-
The Nerves sit ceremonious, like Tombs-
The stiff Heart questions was it He, that bore,
And Yesterday or Centuries before?

The feet, mechanical, go round-
Of Ground, or Air, or Ought-
A Wooden way
Regardless grown,
A Quartz contentment like a stone-

This is the Hour of Lead-
Remembered, if outlived,
As Freezing persons, recollect the Snow-
First—Chill—Then Stupor—then the letting go-

—Emily Dickinson, 1862

Mom has been in the nursing home three years now. She is living a very simple life. Remember Thoreau's admonition to "Simply, simplify, simplify." Well, she does. She eats and sleeps and goes to the activity room. I wheel her around the facility. She is usually asleep, groaning like a mourning dove, or sucking on her middle fingers with the ferocity of a starved infant.

She is kept clean with a hammock dip in a large tub. Her clothes are clean every day. Sometimes, her clothes are changed several times a day if her diaper leaks or if she spills food. If she appears cold, someone puts a lap blanket over her. Someone always anticipates her needs. All residents are treated as special and called by name and talked to directly with eye-to-eye contact, just like at Ruby's place.

Local school children visit her and she is always present for sing-a-longs, choir productions, animal visits, and other activities. She even holds the baby goats which are brought regularly by a farmer in the area. She loves them.

Carrie, the Activities Director, is a jolly, exuberant person who spreads joy. She sends a monthly calendar of activities to family members and invites us to join in. She writes a weekly column in the local paper to keep the community informed about the "liveliness" of the home. She is a major factor in the success of the nursing home.

Whenever I visit, I am warmly greeted by the staff. Staff members hold regular care conferences to discuss Mom's "progress." They are very genuine in their caring. As a result, I feel comfortable being here. I don't even fill out the visitors' book because I don't feel like a visitor.

There are times when I hold Mom's milk shake while she sucks it through a straw. Other times, I feed her ice cream which she seems to enjoy. She's like a baby bird with her mouth open after every swallow. I regularly cut her hair in a short style and frequently brush her hair, not because it needs it, but because she seems to be comforted by the brushing. I bring new clothing to Mom from time to time. Mom seems to like it when I rub her back.

Mom's days are regulated. Meals are on time. She's fed pureed foods by me or an aide. She has medication to control scratching. She is safe. She participates in simple pleasures and she shows no evidence of pain. She seems content. She is surrounded by love.

She is clearly in the final stage of Alzheimer's disease, but she has some strengths. She can indicate her awareness of food by actions (spitting out, swallowing, etc.). She can indicate anger when frustrated. She can lift her head and follow a moving object with her eyes at times. She can smile in response to another's smile. She can roll from side to side. She has a startle reflex when there is a loud sound or a sudden movement. She has a grasping reflex. When you put your finger in her hand, she'll grasp it. She has a sucking reflex. If you put a straw or a nipple in her mouth, she'll suck on it. She has a rooting reflex which means that you touch the top, bottom, or sides of Mom's mouth, she'll move her lips in the direction of the stroking.

I mention these strengths because I learned long ago, after assessing critically-ill newborn babies in a neonatal intensive care nursery, that it is important to describe what a baby can do. There are a lot of things the baby can't do, but developmental intervention is based on what the baby can do and go forward from there. The same is true for school children and for you and me. I would rather be assessed on what I can do.

Well, Mom is moving in reverse. The strengths I mentioned are strengths of a newborn baby or a very young infant. That is her stage of development at this time. She's moving toward death. The end is, in some ways, like the beginning.

30

She Has Been a Blessing

They say that "Time Assuages"-
Time never did assuage-
An actual suffering strengthens
As Sinews do—with age-

Time is a Test of Trouble-
But not a Remedy-
If such it prove, it prove too
There was no Malady-

—Emily Dickinson, 1863

When I look back over the years of caring for Mom, I realize that she has been a blessing, not only during my growing up years, but during these past eleven years down the Alzheimer's path.

I have, finally, been blessed with real patience and peace. I can answer the same question put to me 20 times or more and no longer feel any rage. I can even laugh about it with other caregivers. I can sit still with Mom as she sleeps without worrying about other things to be done. She has taught me to be still and enjoy the moment. After all, that's all we have. According to Loretta Lariat, "Yesterday is history. Tomorrow is a mystery. Today is a gift. That's why it is called the present." Mom has given me a gift, my "now".

The small crises which occurred, like Mom's broken arm and hip, her itch and sudden hospital discharge have taught me that I can handle a crisis. This was an important lesson when Dick, my husband of 40 years, died suddenly of an abdominal aneurysm. I was devastated. I thought Alzheimer's disease was the worst thing. It isn't. I went to the nursing home to tell Mom about Dick's death. Her eyes were vacant and she nodded off as I wept. I felt empty and at a loss for something to take away my profound pain. I missed not only Dick, but my Mom.

Because of Mom, I had retired and Dick had retired later. Dick and I had a year of 24 hour togetherness, something I will always treasure. Without Mom's illness, we both would still have been working.

Because Dick frequently went to the nursing home, he had developed many friendships with the residents. He would hold their frail or arthritic hands and it seemed as if he gave them strength. His true gentle nature was returned in kind.

In lieu of flowers for Dick's funeral, we asked that donations go to the nursing home. Through the generosity of those he touched in his life, many things were purchased including a new patio set and a camera. In the activity room is a Redlin print with a plaque which reads, In memory of Dick Swanson for his kindness and generosity." So, every time I visit, I am reminded of Dick. It's a good feeling.

Mom was usually physically fit during her life and during the majority of her Alzheimer's disease. Dick had often said, "She'll outlive me." She did.

I was blessed by the Alzheimer's experience because I knew I was not alone. My family surrounded me with love and support. I joined a support group for my new path without Dick. He and I had a very special loving relationship and I needed help in dealing with his loss. I realized that I probably would have needed a support group to deal with the Alzheimer's if I hadn't had Dick. He always had a willing ear, gave sage advice, and offered loving acceptance. I didn't have that anymore. I was not able to deal with Alzheimer's and with Dick's death. In my support group, I was able to say, "I am needy." I was able to sob openly and receive support. Most importantly, I was able to be with people who had lost a loved one and who understood.

I used to say, "I don't know how people deal with Alzheimer's alone". Now, I was alone. Now, I know that no one has to do it alone especially with a close family like mine and good friends. For those who don't have close friends or family, there are support groups. The Alzheimer's Association is an excellent source for resources.

A trauma such as AD in a family can tear a family apart or it can bring it closer. When family members join together to support each other, the feelings of helplessness and lack of control are shared and emotional ties are strengthened. My brother showed no interest and did not join with me to care for Mom. This was a huge disappointment. I felt even more helpless and angry. My family bore the cost of Mom's care without his help. His lack of action and support severed our ties.

My grown children were a constant presence in Mom's declining years and a precious emotional support for me as a caregiver. Somehow, this experience has taught us that we can trust each other with our lives. I had Mom's Power of Attorney and my children have mine. We have learned that love doesn't end…even with Alzheimer's disease and death.

I learned that I rarely use the lessons learned from my Doctoral program (unless they are humility and persistence), but I frequently use the lessons I learned from Mom. My initial reaction to a new crisis may be dismay, but I take a deep breath and prepare myself for a new path. I know that it means I'm going to grow. I'm going to learn.

I learned a lot about nutrition. A balanced diet is important for good health. I learned ways to compensate for Mom's poor appetite. She ate like a bird. Remember the mourning dove!

I learned about friends. Real friends understand that giving care is exhausting and leaves little time for get-togethers or phone calls. Real friends call occasionally and ask you over even when you don't have the energy to reciprocate. Our close friends, Bill, Barb, Vito, Margie, Athy, Brooke, Jini, Don, and Virginia called us and were good listeners. These are friends I have known for more than fifty years and they are, along with our family, the treasures of a long life. Dick used to say, "You're wealthy if you have friends." We are wealthy in that way.

I learned that it is okay to feel rage and resentment about the situation. Sharing these feelings helps to diffuse them. Deciding ahead of time how I was going to deal with the rage helped. I learned to meditate or relax with deep breaths and eyes closed. Over time, rage and resentment gave way to acceptance and understanding, a sense of peace about a situation.

I developed other new ways for dealing with a crisis. I was comforted by the thought, "This, too, shall pass" and pass it did. I no longer feel anger in being a caregiver. I feel privileged that I am capable of helping Mom in her final years. As George Bernard Shaw said, "I want to be used up when I die, for the harder I work, the more I live. Life is no brief candle to me, it is sort of splendid torch which I have got hold of for a moment, and I want to make it burn as brightly as possible before handing it on to future generations".

With caregiving, one is challenged to be "used up." There were many days when I felt "used up", but those were days when I was intensely alive. I never thought I would feel this way. Mom and her condition have been lovingly integrated into our family.

I was blessed by knowing the residents in the nursing home who have lived interesting lives and would sometimes share them with me if I sat down next to them long enough and often enough to become their friend. The wisdom from a long life experience of the elderly gave me new insights.

I've been blessed with humility. I was never a "Wonder Woman." I could never do it all. I found that it wasn't healthy to try to do it all. My limitations were not failures. They just were limitations and that was okay. Sometimes, I was able to overcome limitations and, if I couldn't, so be it. It's okay. I'm human.

I learned that the path I chose to take was my way. Other people have their ways to deal with Alzheimer's and it's just as good or bad or, perhaps, better than my path. I don't judge others because it's not helpful and we can never know what is in someone else's head and heart. We are all in a similar struggle. We must be patient with ourselves. We are all human.

I learned a lot about Alzheimer's disease. When I meet someone who has a loved one with AD, I am drawn to them. I know that deep within them is a core of pain. I also know that they have shifted priorities and usually know what's important in life. They are not superficial. I am drawn to them as I was when I worked with parents of handicapped children, not out of pity, but out of admiration that they are surviving and, yes, even thriving. And yes, they understand because they've "been there." I understand because I've "been there."

H. Thurman captures the feeling:

> I share with you the agony of your grief, the anguish of your heart finds echo in my own. I know I cannot enter all you feel nor bear with you the burden of your pain; I can but offer what my love does give: the strength of caring, the warmth of one who seeks to understand the silent storm-swept barrenness of so great a loss. This I do in quiet ways, that on your lonely path you may not walk alone.

I have learned ways of responding to Mom in each stage on her path. Sheila Kane King said it best:

> If your loved one is in the early stages, savor your conversations, and let them reminisce. You will cherish those times in the days ahead.

> If you are struggling through the middle stages, listen to those you love,
> And, if they tell you to give up your loved one to professional care, give it some serious thought. Children should not have to lose both parents.

And if you are in the final stages of this devastating illness, take solace that when it is over, it becomes possible to remember her as she was before, and good memories are a great and unexpected gift.

I flow with life now, sometimes with a lack of understanding, but always with the belief that I can meet life's challenges. I am a survivor until death comes. I will make my life, what's left of it, part of Mom's and Dick's legacy. This book is part of that legacy. I want people to know the blessings as well as the horrors of Alzheimer's disease. I want caregivers to know they are not alone. I want researchers to know the ups and downs that caregivers face so that the researchers will realize the urgency for a cure.

I have a new understanding of meaning in life. Emily Dickinson, my favorite poet, wrote in 1864:

> If I can stop one heart from breaking
> I shall not live in vain
> If I can ease one Life the aching
> Or cool one Pain
>
> Or help one fainting Robin
> Unto his Nest again
> I shall not live in Vain.

I have helped a mourning dove to find peace. I want to continue to be a part of a healing community such as Hospice or facilitate a support group. Mom has given me a new life direction and with it, new meaning.

Finally, I learned that I have a humanity that makes me proud. I can love someone when they give me nothing in return...yet everything. Sherwin B. Nuland in *How We Die,* states, "If there is wisdom to be found, it must be in the knowledge that human beings are capable of the kind of love and loyalty that transcends not only the physical debasement but even the spiritual weariness of the years of sorrow."

I learned that I am capable of unconditional love, a love that transcends all others. I feel this love for my children and grandchildren. They can rest assured that, no matter what, they are loved, unconditionally. Yes. Mom, I got my reward. You were right.

No wonder we do not lose heart! Though our outward humanity is in decay yet day by day we are inwardly renewed. Our troubles are slight and short-lived;

and their outcome an eternal glory which outweighs them by far. Meanwhile our eyes are fixed not on the things that are seen, but on things that are unseen; for what is seen passes away; what is unseen is eternal.

St. Paul, 11 Corinthians 4, 17, 18

31

The Ripening

I held a Jewel in my fingers-
And went to sleep-
The day was warm, and the winds were prosy-
I said "'Twill keep"-

I woke—and chid my honest fingers,
The Gem was gone-
And now, an Amethyst remembrance
Is all I own-

—Emily Dickinson, 1861

Mom died in late summer just three weeks before her 93rd birthday after 11 years with Alzheimer's disease and a year and a half after Dick's death. Just before her death, she was unable to walk or talk, feed herself, eat solid foods, or keep her eyes open. She had no bladder or bowel control. A month before her death, I noticed some changes. She lost more weight, ate even less of the pureed food, and slept most of the time. Her eyes were rarely open even when awake. Because of her sleeping, she was in bed most of the time. I mention these things that she can't or doesn't do because caregivers ask me what the final stage is like. What Mom could do before she died was to sleep, breathe with difficulty, and occasionally open her eyes.

I sensed that her body was ready to be released. I asked, at a care conference at the nursing home before she died, if Hospice services would be appropriate. I asked for two reasons. I had attended the Hospice support group sessions when Dick died and the people and support were wonderful. I also asked because I needed confirmation that Mom was near to death. I was asked, "What could Hospice services do that we are not doing?" Well, she was receiving good care.

She didn't need medication for pain. She seemed peaceful. The matter was dropped.

No one confirmed that death was near for Mom. That would be one value of Hospice services, acknowledgement that Mom was near death. The Hospice program also provides bereavement services. This includes follow-up counseling for the survivor or survivors. Without Hospice, only one person followed up on me. That was Marge.

Marge, the night supervisor, was an exemplary nurse. She was very professional and caring. She took a personal interest in each resident. She clearly respected them. She was a source of great comfort to the families of residents. Marge called and said, "Jennie, your Mom's chin is cold. It's not a good sign. I thought you might want to come and be with her". Marge helped me by acknowledging the seriousness of Mom's condition. I had a feeling, by the tone of Marge's voice that Mom was near death.

I rushed over to the nursing home and sat with Mom for hours. Her oxygen level was low. Her breathing was slightly labored. She was given oxygen and her level returned to normal. Then she slept peacefully. The Activities Director and the Social Worker brought me lemonade, cookies, and hugs.

I spent the days with Mom during her last week of life. I held her hand, brushed her hair, rubbed her arms, legs, and back. I told her "I love you" over and over. I read passages from the Bible to her. I found the quiet time with Mom oddly comforting. Dick died so quickly, I didn't have time to say good-bye. I had time now to say good-bye. It's as Frank and Ginny Maier stated in *A Second Chance at Life:*

> "Love isn't just for the good times; eventually it means having to share someone else's pain. That's when you no longer take it for granted, but know love for what it is: a gift freely given".

I also spent time reviewing my life and hers. My thoughts were often of Dick and my "Winds of Yesterday."

Friday morning, I dressed, had coffee and a bagel, and drove to the nursing home. I saw Mom stretched out on the bed without a blanket. The frailness of her body saddened and shocked me. I learned later that she weighed 64 pounds. She made a gasping sound with each breath. She had the gray-white pallor of death. I kissed her and her chin and nose were cold.

I sat with her all day. I ran home at dinner time to quickly call my children. While I was gone, an aide tried to feed solid food to Mom. When I returned, a nurse approached me and said, "I was just going to call you. She did eat some dinner but she doesn't look good now."

The sun is slowly setting, just like Mom. I held her hand and we sat in quietness. I was in awe of the significance of her passing. I had an awareness of the spiritual power of these moments. It seemed as if the entire world was quiet. I felt an emptiness in my gut.

Then, a nurse came in and started suctioning Mom's throat. The spell was broken. She said, "It will help her breathing. The food might have gone down the wrong way". As she took the tube and placed it in Mom's throat, Mom seemed very distressed. The nurse kept suctioning her throat, pulling the tube in and out, in and out. I didn't think she knew that Mom was dying. Mom's arms were moving in a jerky fashion. Finally, I said, "No More." The suctioning stopped. Mom's breathing was not improved. I was sorry that Mom was disturbed in her passing. The nurse left.

I put Mom's head higher up under a pillow and held both of her hands. I said, "Mom, let's say a prayer. Now I lay me down to sleep..." This seems more appropriate for Mom than the Lord's Prayer. When the prayer was over, Mom's breathing slowed. Two nurses came in. Mom raised her head slightly and opened her eyes for the first time in two weeks. She looked right at me with wide haunting eyes. One nurse said, "She's saying good-bye to you" but I knew the sign.

> The eyes glaze once-and that is Death-
> Impossible to feign
> The Beads upon the Forehead
> By homely Anguish strung.

—Emily Dickinson, 1861
(Excerpt from "I Like a look of Agony")

Then, Mom laid her head down to the side. A yellow liquid ran out of her mouth and down the sheets. Her eyes were closed. Her face felt cold. Her body was still. Mom was ready for her harvest.

The nurses, the Activity Director, and the new Social Worker came in and hugged me. Some had tears in their eyes. Then, they left me for a quiet time. I hugged and kissed Mom for the last time. My tears fell on her face. I had been preparing for this day for years, but it is still a shock. After all, she was my Mom.

The doctor on duty confirmed her death. Mom has been dying with open eyes for eleven years. Only now, death is finally confirmed.

Everyone thinks that when he gets it, it's going to be quick, splendid, and with just a dab of heroism. No one ever thinks he is going to be nibbled away".

From *Going Gently* by Robert Downs

That's it. Mom's life has slowly been nibbled away. She has been dying to live. I am glad that she died in her "home" and not in a hospital. I have confidence that she is heaven-bound. Emily Dickinson wrote "I Never Saw a Moor" (1865):

> I never saw a moor-
> I never saw the Sea-
> Yet know I how the Heather looks
> And what a Billow be.
>
> I never spoke with God,
> Not visited in heaven-
> Yet certain am I of the spot
> As if the checks were given-

Suddenly I remembered the brain autopsy. I needed to make arrangements because the autopsy had to take place within 12 hours after death. I called the funeral home director. He said he would be at the nursing home in 30 minutes. I had previously made arrangements for him to transport Mom to the Medical Center 50 miles away. I was grateful that he was available because it was late on a Friday evening. I had to run home to get the form for the autopsy and send a telegram to the doctor at the medical Center giving my approval for the autopsy. I called several surrounding towns and was unable to find a telegraph office which was open.

In desperation, I called my daughter Laurie and asked her if she could find a telegraph office in the Chicago area as soon as possible. I hoped an office will be open there. Laurie called back in a few minutes. She sent the telegram. She always comes through when needed.

I called my sons and jumped back in the car. I had to give the autopsy forms to the funeral director to give to the Medical Center. Halfway back to the nursing home, the car stopped. I sat by the side of the road in the darkness. I said a prayer. I turned on the ignition. The car started.

My children and grandchildren arrived late Saturday morning. Meanwhile, I made the funeral arrangements as well as arrangements to have Mom's body transported, after the funeral, to Georgia for burial next to Dad. We made a photo album of Mom's life for the services.

> The Bustle in a House
> The Morning after Death
> Is solemnest of industries
> Enacted upon Earth-
>
> The Sweeping up the Heart
> And putting Love away
> We shall not want to use again
> Until Eternity.

—Emily Dickinson, 1866

The Pastor who ministered to Mom while she was at the nursing home for three years conducted the service. He lifted our spirits as he talked about Mom and her harvest. He and his wife sang Mom's favorite song, "You are My Sunshine". Our close friends made the two hour journey for the funeral. No one from the nursing home was at the service. This was a disappointment. Ruby was there. My brother's daughter was present. My brother didn't come. He did, however, oversee her burial arrangements in her hometown in Georgia.

The funeral director did a wonderful job preparing Mom's body for viewing. She looked like mom of long ago. I was thankful for this last memory. Mom seemed to have transcended the indignities of Alzheimer's disease. She had dignity in death that mirrored her life before the disease. There was no sign of an autopsy as you looked at Mom's head.

My grandson, Blake, read a poem about death which Mom had given me when my Dad died. The poem mentioned death as a transition and not an ending. My son, Scott, read a short biography Mom had written many years earlier. She had a full and productive life.

Laurie read a piece which she had written before Mom's death about her Grandma titled, "I'm Fighting":

> I'm fighting, fighting to remember
> Grandma-
> Pill box hats and French twists with lady friends,
> Tea with Eleanor Roosevelt,

Paintings, delicate on china,
Travels by train with Ches,
Life and family in southern Georgia.
Wonderful stories.
Wonderful life.

I'm fighting, fighting to remember
Grandma-
A sugary sweet Southern lady
Full of happiness, energy, gone…
Not dead, but gone.
Robbed of dignity and self.
No more stories to tell,
No more adventures to pursue,
No more reason to live.

I'm fighting, fighting to remember
Grandma-
Before Alzheimer's took its wicked course,
Now…skin covers bones
Muscles long atrophied
Eyes vacant
Hair lacking luster
Body curled in a fetal position
Fingers being sucked with the ferocity of a newborn babe.

I'm fighting, fighting to remember
Grandma-
Small build, enormous heart,
Please go, I pray,
Please find your peace,
"Be sweet", she'd say,
"I love you", I reply.

Hats, tea, paintings, stories,
I'm fighting, fighting.

—Laurie Swanson Kiesewetter, 1995

There was not a dry eye in the place when Laurie read this.

I follow up with "Cleo." I wrote this because I wanted everyone to remember Mom as she was before Alzheimer's.

A Southern Belle
Born in the land of the kudzu
In a house with five siblings
Daughter of the town builder
Growing up with promenades, white gloves, and stockings
Eating Talmadge hams and pot liquor with cornbread
A carefree youth in a loving family
An artist painting on canvas and china
A teacher giving hope in the slums of Foggy Bottom
A mother, always loving, rubbing backs
A wife, happily married for 53 years
A staunch Christian singing, "In the Garden"
A grandmother telling everybody, "They're mine"
A Great-Grandmother kissing hands and saying, "Be sweet"
An Alzheimer's victim-loving everyone, knowing no one
A special person who was greatly loved.

We went to a restaurant for a meal after the funeral to celebrate Mom's life. Because of death, we are more aware of the precious moments of life, the dash between birth and death.

Death will greet me, too.
Until then, I live.
Her legacy, I accept.
The more I have to give.

32

The Promise of Death is Life

Time does go on-
I tell it gay to those who suffer now-
They shall survive-
There is a sun-
They don't believe it now.

—Emily Dickinson, 1868

According to *Augustine, City of God*, Book 3, Chapter 10:

"As doctors, when they examine the state of a patient and recognize that Death is at hand, pronounce 'He is dying, he will not recover'. So we must say from the moment a man is born: "He will not recover.""

Life is always fatal. At some point, all of us will not recover. I remember a very caring psychiatrist tending to a dying patient who said, "Doctor, I'm dying." Softly and reverently, she responded, "I am too. I just don't know when and how." This is true for most of us, but death is true for all of us. Kazantrakis writes:

It is not morbid to think of death. It is morbid never to think of death! Life without Death is morbid, for it is an empty life, a dead life. When anything becomes truly a matter of life or death to you, only then do you truly appreciate it; only then do you give it your whole attention; only then do you give it life.

I remember back to special moments when I was gripped with fear like the time Dick arrived home four hours late after a blinding snowstorm. His life was paramount in my thoughts during the vigil. He was pleasantly overwhelmed by my welcome when he arrived home exhausted. Then, there was the time that my grandson, Blake, fell off of a pier and floated momentarily until his father jumped in to rescue him. I am still haunted by the image of his blonde hair floating in the water. These kinds of moments make me realize the vulnerability of life as well as the preciousness of life. Dick's death made me confront the inevitability of death, a natural part of life, but his loss pains me still.

Why can't we view life as if we are ripening? The ripening process begins from the moment of conception and continues throughout life. We grow and develop or ripen. Meridel LeSueur reminds us that things in nature do not age. They ripen. She describes the cycle of the natural world in a sunflower metaphor of seed time, ripening, and harvesting. Cato Major de senectute, 44 B.C.E., related:

> "…just as apples when they are green are with difficulty plucked from the tree, but when ripe and mellow fall of themselves, so, with the young, death comes as the result of force while with the old it is the result of ripeness. To me, indeed, the thought of this 'ripeness' for death is so pleasant, that the nearer I approach death the more I feel like one is in sight of land at last and is about to anchor in his home port after a long voyage."

The ripening may lead to peace, serenity, comfort, and contentment for some people as they approach death. I saw this in Mom at the end. She has finally ripened. It has been a long journey. She has spent a lot of time in the waiting room, slowly dying with eyes open. I often prayed that medical science would not intervene to cause over-ripeness or rot.

Martin Grotjahn writes in "The Day I Got Old" (1982):

> I don't work anymore. I don't walk anymore. Peculiarly enough, I feel well about it. I sit in the sun watching the falling leaves slowly sail across the swimming pool. I think, I dream, I draw, I sit-I feel free of worry-almost free of this world of reality. If anyone had told me I would be quietly happy just sitting here reading a little, writing a little, and enjoying life in a quiet and modest way, I, of course, would not have believed. That a walk across the street to the corner of the park satisfies me when I always thought a four-hour walk was just not good enough: that surprises me.

His statement causes me to reflect on Mom's hours looking out the window. She seemed to be quietly peaceful with her "Winds of Yesterday." We might think of the elderly as in a unique cycle of ripening, the preparation for the harvest. They need the right conditions. Just as apple trees need pruning, the person with Alzheimer's needs a simplified environment, a cutting back. Just as special care is needed for roses, such as insect spraying, fertilizer, and protection from the cold, so too, does the Alzheimer's person need special conditions to flower and to experience life's harvest.

Mom and I traveled a long path for eleven years and I believe that we are both at peace. The nurses said of Mom in the last few months, "She seems content." I never thought I would hear that. Mom no longer made the sound of the mourning dove.

Over her eleven years with Alzheimer's disease, Mom was slowly dying. Her brain cells were dying. Her brain was shrinking. She was losing her self slowly and relentlessly. We must mobilize our resources to find a cause for this disease so that we have "a world without Alzheimer's disease."

Dick's death, to me, was like a green apple plucked before time. But, judging from the positive impact he had on the lives of family and friends and the love surrounding his memory, there was a ripening and Dick is enjoying his harvest.

I think Mom completed her ripening and we both can look forward to the harvest, some of which I have already experienced. Mom is now free of her disease. Death is the only cure at this time.

Because of Mom and Dick, I will live more abundantly, not with material things, but with memories and love which nourish the soul forever. Mom left me with another major benefit.

I now know that the promise of death is life.

THE END

Epilogue

It has been many years since Mom died. A lot has happened in my life since then. Caregiving, whether in the home, or in a nursing home, or in a CBRF, was a totally absorbing experience for me. I rarely read a whole book, went to a play or concert, or really had fun. Life is serious when you are a caregiver.

It took me a while to adjust to life without Mom. It took me a long time to adjust to life without Dick. His death was so sudden and unexpected. I didn't have time to say good-bye. My grief over Dick's death was more complicated because I was in the process of anticipatory grieving of Mom's upcoming death.

I have finally forgiven my brother because I do not walk in his shoes.

With the help of family and friends, I am a caregiver-survivor of Alzheimer's disease and not a caregiver-victim. Mom always said that I would get my reward someday. Today, I am happily married to Tom. He is my reward for loving.

Tom and I are volunteers for Hospice as facilitators of support groups for people who are grieving. Our blessings continue.

During the time of Mom's Alzheimer's disease and Dick's death, I never thought I could be happy again.

I am.

There's always hope.

Mom's Autopsy Results

Mom's brain weighed 1060 grams. The average brain weighs 1500 grams. It is common for the brain weight to be below average because of the loss of tissue and cells. The weight of Mom's body at death was 64 pounds.

The dura matter is the membrane that sheathes the brain. It was pale grey, finely granular, and glistening. The meninges or membranes were thin, semi-transparent, and finely granular. The surface of the brain showed slight atrophy of the gyri and slight widening of the sulci. No gross abnormalities of the cranial nerves were seen.

There was a slight thinning of the cortex and a slight enlargement of the ventricles. When the brain shrinks, the ventricles naturally grow.

The impression was cerebral atrophy.

The microscopic description indicated a slight to moderate loss of neurons and gliosis in the cortex. The characteristic plaques and tangles were seen. Some senile plaques are normal in an aging brain. In people older than 75 years of age, there is an average of 8.2 senile plaques per microscopic field. Mom had higher counts in the hippocampus, mid frontal lobes, Wernicke's area, and the superior temporal lobes.

The cerebellum and brain stem were unremarkable. There was no evidence of Pick's disease or Lewy body disease (other types of dementia).

The diagnosis was Alzheimer's disease, mild in degree. The mild fits the standard criteria used in autopsies. It usually has nothing to do with the patient's symptoms. Usually, the longer the person has Alzheimer's disease, the more severe the symptoms.

One half of the brain was sent to a medical center for a biochemical analysis. No results are available because the patients are not identified for the study.

Index to the First Lines of Emily Dickinson's Poems

*Johnson, Thomas H. (Editor), *The Complete Poems of Emily Dickinson,* Little, Brown and Company, Boston, 1890, 1891, 1896 by Roberts, 1914, 1918, 1919, 1924, 1929, 1932, 1935, 1937, 1942, by Martha Dickinson Bianchi, 1951, 1955, by the President and Fellows of Harvard College. 1952 by Alfred Leete Hampton, 1957, 1958, 1960 by M.L. Hampson.

References

AARP (American Association of Retired Persons)
601 E. St., N.W., Washington, D.C. 20049
202-434-2277 or 800-424-3410 www.aarp.org

ADEAR (Alzheimer's Disease Education and Referral Center),
P.O. Box 8250, Silver Spring, MD. 20907-8250
301-495-3311 or 800-438-4380 www.alzheimers.org/adear

Alzheimer's Association, National Headquarters,
919 N. Michigan Avenue, Suite 1100, Chicago, Il. 60611-1676
312-335-8700 or 800-272-3900, www.alz.org

Downs, Robert, *Going Gently. N.Y.,*. Bobbs-Merrill, *1973*.

Frankl, Viktor E.. *Man's Search for Meaning.* Boston, MA, Beacon Press, 1959.

Grotjahn, Martin, "The Day I Got Old". *Psychiatric Clinics of North America, 1982.*

Havel, Vaclav, *Disturbing The Peace: A Conversation with Karel Huizdala.* N.Y., Vintage Books: a division of Random House, Inc., 1991

Johnson, Thomas H., *The Complete Poems of Emily Dickinson.* Boston, NY, and London, Little, Brown and Company, 1960.

Kazantrakis, Nikos, *The Odyssey, A Modern Sequel.* Trans. Kimon Friar. Book 18. N.Y. Simon and Schuster, 1958

Kraeft, Peter J., *Love is Stronger Than Death.* New York, Harper and Row, Publishers, 1979.

Mace, Nancy L. and Robins, Peter V., *The 36 Hour Day: A Family Guide to Caring for Persons with Alzheimer's Illnesses and Memory Loss in Later Life.*

McCowin, Diane Friel, *Living in the Labyrinth: A Personal Journey Through the Maze of Alzheimer's*. New York, A Delta Book published by Dell Publishing, a division of Bantam Doubleday Dell Publishing Group, Inc. 1993.

"Metlife Market Survey of Nursing Home and Home Care Costs", Executive Summary. Westport CT. Metlife Mature Market Institute. Sept., 2004.

Myers, Edward, *When Parents Die: A Guide for Adults*. N.Y. Viking Press, 1983.

National Hospice and Palliative Care Organization
1700 Diagonal Road, Suite 625
Alexander, VA 22314
703-837-1500 www.nhpco.org

Petersen, M.D., Ph.D., Ronald, Editor, *Mayo Clinic on Alzheimer's Disease*. Rochester, MN, Mayo Clinic Health Information. 2002.

Safford, Florence, *Caring for the Mentally Impaired Elderly: A Family Guide*. New York, Henry Holt and Company, 1987.

Shankle, M.S., M.D., Wm. Rodman, and Amen, M.D., Daniel G., *Preventing Alzheimer's: Ways to Help Prevent, Detect, and Even Halt Alzheimer's Disease and Other Forms of Memory Loss*. New York, G.P. Putnam's Sons. 2004

Shenk, David, *The Forgetting: Alzheimer's: Portrait of an Epidemic. Anchor, 2003*.

Snowden, David "Testimony of Dr. David Snowdon" presented to the Subcommittee on Labor, Health, and Human Services, and Education and Related Agencies Committee on Appropriations. Professor in the Dept. of Neurology and the Sanders-Brown Center on Aging at the University of Kentucky, Lexington, KY. March, 2004

Shriver, Maria, *What's Happening to Grandpa*. Boston and New York, Little, Brown and Company and Warner Books. 2004

Thoreau, Henry David, (Journal)

Whitman, Walt, *Selections from Leaves of Grass*. New York, Avenel Books: a division of Crown Publishers, Inc. MCMLXI.

About the Author

Jennie Swanson Dincecco, Ed.D., was the caregiver for her mother who had Alzheimer's disease for eleven years. Dr. Dincecco has a Doctorate in Human Growth and Development and was an Assistant Professor of Pediatrics in a major medical center, as well as the Director of Special Services for the Handicapped in a public school system. Prior to that, she was a Psychoeducational Diagnostician, an elementary and early childhood educator, and the Director of Early Childhood Education in a public school system.

Dr. Dincecco completed her Bachelor of Science at Northwestern University, and a Master of Science and a Doctorate in Human Growth and Development at Northern Illinois University. She has received advanced training in neuropsychology.

Dr. Dincecco has been listed in *Distinguished Leaders in Health Care*, *Who's Who in America*, *Who's Who in the World*, *Who's Who in American Education*, *Who's Who in Medicine and Healthcare*, Who's *Who in International Education*, *and Who's Who in Child Development*. Dr. Dincecco was the recipient of a foreign scholarship from Delta Kappa Gamma (honorary education society). She is an accomplished speaker and has presented seminars to professional and lay audiences throughout the United States and in Scotland.

Dr. Dincecco lives with her husband in Woodstock, Illinois. She is the proud mother of her blended family of four children and the proud grandmother of eleven grandchildren.

Index

0-595-34054-7